RECIPES
FOR
BETTER
BONES

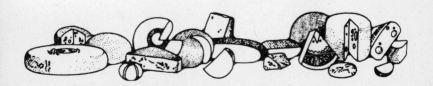

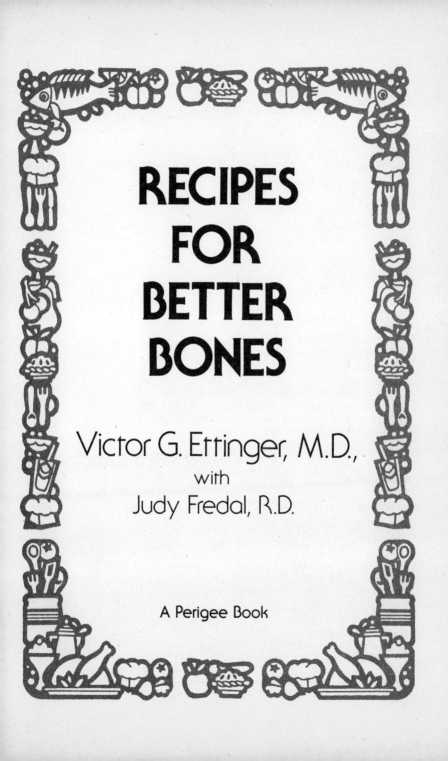

RECIPES FOR BETTER BONES

Victor G. Ettinger, M.D.,
with
Judy Fredal, R.D.

A Perigee Book

This book is dedicated to my wife and daughters and to the other women I know, or will come to know, as patients and as friends.

—VGE

Perigee Books
are published by
The Putnam Publishing Group
200 Madison Avenue
New York, NY 10016

Library of Congress Cataloging-in-Publication Data

Ettinger, Victor G.
  Recipes for better bones.

  "A Perigee book."
  Bibliography: p.
  Includes index.
  1. High-calcium diet—Recipes. 2. Osteoporosis—Prevention.
I. Fredal, Judy II. Title.
RM237.56.E78 1987   641.5'63   87–7262
ISBN 0–399–51401–5

Book design: ARLENE GOLDBERG
Printed in the United States of America
1 2 3 4 5 6 7 8 9 10

CONTENTS

ACKNOWLEDGMENTS

Many people, both professional and lay, contributed to the factual content of this book. To list them individually would court the disaster of forgetting one, so we will just thank them en masse: *Thank you.*

In addition, I specifically want to thank Adrienne Ingrum and Anton Mueller from The Putnam Publishing Group, whose attention to the important details made this book happen; and Anna Jardine, whose copyediting makes the words flow like music. Finally I wish to adjoin the mandatory thanks to my family for putting up with my seclusion for long hours in my study while I wrote and revised this manuscript.

And with sincere thanks and appreciation to Theresa and Francis Fredal, Charlene Muranaka, Nancy Ingram, Maria Cardinale and Patty Hall for help in recipe development and testing; Jennifer Mack, Chris Kimball, Meegan Earl, Vicki Fernandez, Beverly DeDonatis, Loretta and Gary Beasley, Barbara and Jose Carrera and Ed Muranaka, our tasters and critics; and Anne Bradford and Rose Mary Popp for their professional assistance. Special thanks to Rayne Pang for his support.

PART I

Information

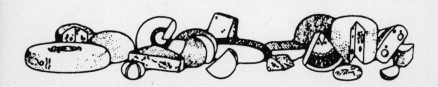

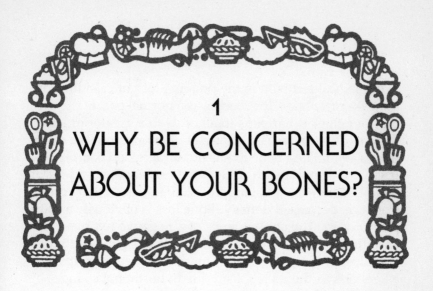

1

WHY BE CONCERNED ABOUT YOUR BONES?

OVERVIEW

Osteoporosis has been known as a disease since the nineteenth century. Even then it was apparent that elderly women had an increased risk of long bone fractures after even minor falls. However, postmenopausal estrogen deficiency was not linked to this disease until early in the twentieth century. How this protective effect of estrogen works is unknown. It is thought to be indirect, probably through effects on other hormones. It is only recently, within the last few decades, that we have become aware that several other hormones—progesterone, androgens, PTH and so on—are also involved in a less significant though still important manner.

What exactly is osteoporosis? In financial terms in the United States, it was a $7.3 billion disease for hip fracture alone in 1983, an increase from $6 billion in 1980, and this

9

is not including the expense for post-hospitalization nursing home care.

In medical terms, it is the ongoing loss of calcium from bones—*osteopenia*—that occurs as a normal part of the process of aging. It happens to all of us to a greater or lesser degree. Osteopenia is a universal phenomenon; the cause of this age-related bone loss is not understood completely. It is very important to differentiate osteopenia, a loss of bone density, from osteoporosis, the disease that results from this decreased density. Bone loss is obviously a complex process, the consequence of a negative net bone balance (less new bone being built while old bone continues to be lost at the usual rate). The process seems to involve alterations in the metabolism due to hormonal changes of aging that interact with bone minerals.

Let us discuss what bone is so that we can have a better idea of what is happening. Bone consists of an organic matrix made up of collagen (strong semi-elastic protein fibers that hold body parts together) and noncollagen proteins, impregnated with calcium and phosphorus. There are two major forms of bone. The outer shell (cortical bone) of a long bone, necessary for support, is strong and compact. This outer part makes up 80% of the bone. The inner part of a bone (trabecular bone) is made up of a series of porous interconnected plates; it is here that the blood vessels and marrow reside. The amount of each kind of bone varies in different bones—spine bones are predominantly trabecular while hip bones have more cortical bone. This difference results in a dissimilar response to the various metabolic influences and a disparate chance of fracture.

Several hormones are involved in the development and maintenance of bone. These include vitamin D (which in spite of its name is not a vitamin, but a hormone), which is made in the skin or ingested in food. This important hormone allows the absorption of dietary calcium and has

several other metabolic functions relative to bone aug-
mentation.

Calcium accumulates in bones up to approximately age
twenty-five. Over the next decade the amount of bone
calcium remains fairly stable. Starting at about thirty-five
years of age a natural, gradual loss of calcium begins. Bone
loss occurs at the rate of approximately 3% per decade,
starting in the mid-thirties. This loss continues slowly; in
women, at the time of menopause (either natural or sur-
gically induced), a marked acceleration of bone loss occurs,
lasting approximately five to seven years. Bone loss then
slows down somewhat but may continue at a rate of up
to 9% per decade until the seventies, then returning to a
more gradual loss until the late seventies, at which time
it becomes imperceptible.

Osteopenia takes place in both sexes but becomes a problem significantly later in males because men start with a
greater bone density. This is probably related to their greater
intake of calcium in their teens and twenties, as well as
the greater amount of physical activity that they usually
undertake. The male hormone testosterone also plays an
ill-defined role. Therefore it takes longer to reach a critically
low mass. It is apparent that the risk of developing osteoporosis in adult life depends on bone mass at maturity.

As we gain more knowledge, it is evident that osteoporosis is not a single disease but can be separated into
several types, differentiated on the basis of fracture pat-
terns and age when bone loss begins. Type I (postmenopausal) osteoporosis most frequently occurs in the trabecular
bone of the spine in women aged fifty-five to seventy-five
and results in vertebral fractures. Type II (involutional or
senile) osteoporosis usually results in hip fractures in both
sexes at an older age and involves the loss of both kinds
of bones. Having one type of osteoporosis does not nec-
essarily indicate the presence of the other. Since osteo-

porosis is a silent disease, we will not know of its presence until a fracture or deformity, with or without trauma, appears. In order for a break to occur, the trauma may be of only minimal degree.

Who is likely to get osteoporosis? If a typical patient can be described, *she* would be a northern European Caucasian over the age of fifty. Blacks are much less prone to problems than are whites. This is certainly due to the fact that blacks start out with denser bones at any age, compared to nonblacks, for unknown reasons. For this same reason, European (and probably Asian) women are at higher risk than African-origin females. The risk for the Latino and other populations at this time is unknown.

In a typical Caucasian ethnic group, 50% of women over age sixty-five will have wedging of the spine—the rectangular bone will be partially collapsed and will develop a triangular shape. This effect shows a steady increase with age. A complete break will cause the spinal bones to look like pancakes. These compression fractures will occur in 10% of Caucasian women by age sixty-five and in 20% by age seventy. In addition, and more serious, 15% will experience hip fracture over their lifetime, with a 2% chance of hip fracture for each year after eighty. Additionally, 15% will have wrist fractures, which can be severely disabling in an elderly individual who may already have significant problems with arthritis. Is this due to genetic, nutritional, environmental or constitutional causes? The question is currently under intensive investigation in the hope that the answer may give medical science a better handle on prevention and treatment.

Thin individuals are known to be more prone to problems than are the overweight. This is probably because of their smaller bone mass; they reach the theoretical fracture threshold faster. The protective effect of obesity is due to the estrogen production that occurs in fat tissue. (This may be the only truly beneficial effect of obesity. Overweight women are, however, at substantially greater risk of uterine cancer because of excess estrogen.) Early menopause or surgical removal of the ovaries without replacement estrogen treatment is also a known cause of osteoporosis. There is some suggestive information indicating that pregnancy and breast-feeding may have a limited protective effect. The reasons for this are entirely unknown.

Men indeed also have an increased risk of osteoporotic fractures, though starting at a significantly later age because of their higher baseline bone density. The overall chance for men of all ages of having a hip or wrist fracture over their lifetime is less than 5%. This is also true of black men or women. This sex difference in bone loss is poorly understood. Be that as it may, the most common fracture in men is that of the hip, followed next by shoulder and pelvis breaks, while in women the most common site is the wrist, then the spine, and then the shoulder, hip and pelvis, in that order. Sex and weight are only two considerations in bone loss. Other contributing factors include a positive family history; low muscle mass resulting from prolonged exercise—muscle mass and muscle activity are correlated with a greater local bone mass until a certain level of exercise is surpassed, and at that point additional activity is unhealthy; the use of diet pills; lack of sunlight, especially in cloudy and overcast countries such as England, and among the frequently home-bound elderly, because of the decreased production of vitamin D in the skin; low-calcium diets, as exemplified by the minimal calcium-containing foods in the typical teenager's diet. Though it is not certain, some evidence suggests the requirements for calcium may actually *increase* with age. A somewhat speculative association is with high-protein diets, which are associated with high loss of calcium in urine. This may be why Eskimos, who eat protein-rich foods, are found to have a high rate of osteoporosis, in spite of their high intake of Vitamin D.

The disease of osteoporosis has its onset in the sixth decade for women and the eighth decade for men. The most prominent factors for its onset at this time include lack of exercise, decreased estrogen for any reason including excessive exercise, prolonged bed rest and inadequate calcium intake as a youth. The use of several different medications as well as nonmedical substances also plays a very significant role. Such drugs as glucocorticoids (cortisonelike substances) block calcium uptake by bones. One of these is Prednisone, which at a relatively low dose of 15 milligrams per day can lead to fractures, especially of the ribs and spine, and degenerative changes in the hip, necessitating total hip replacement.

Nicotine from smoking leads to less dense bones partly because smokers tend to be thinner than nonsmokers and women smokers undergo menopause earlier (for some women maybe this is a benefit of smoking?); in addition, nicotine has a yet undetermined direct effect on bone metabolism. Other frequently used dietary components that contribute to a significantly increased risk of developing the disease are caffeinated drinks including coffee and colas, which are becoming archenemies of good health, and the known toxic chemical alcohol. Heparin, a drug used to dissolve blood clots, and methotrexate, a frequently used anticancer medication that is now being used for other chronic degenerative diseases, are also known culprits.

Several less documented causes for osteoporosis include high-protein diets (possibly because more calcium is bound preventing its absorption); and poorly controlled diabetes mellitus, which is associated with an increased ankle-fracture rate, rather uncommon in the nondiabetic. Rheumatoid arthritis may also be a cause, possibly secondary, as a result of treatment with cortisonelike drugs. It is interesting to note that osteoporosis is not increased in osteoarthritis, a much more commonly encountered joint problem; in actual fact it may be decreased.

A serious cause of osteoporosis is the use of thyroid hormone in greater than replacement doses; like the disease of hyperthyroidism, this may lead to excessive loss of bone. It is critical that early treatment be instituted because once the bone is lost, there is no return of this lost bone. It is now standard practice to get patients out of bed as soon after surgery as possible, since immobilization leads rapidly, after only a few weeks, to consequential bone loss.

Osteomalacia, the effect of vitamin D deficiency on bones, in the elderly is frequently associated with osteoporosis because of vitamin D deficiency from low intake, low sun exposure, deficiency in metabolism from liver or kidney disease, alcoholism and use of some antacids that bind phosphate. These usually contain aluminum, and it is important to be aware of this since the ingestion of antacids is very common in the elderly. Fortunately, a deficit of vitamin D is easily treatable with supplements.

The following diseases or disorders are also associated with increased bone-thinning and risk of fracture: Cushing's syndrome, from excess cortisone production; prolactin excess due to either a tumor or pituitary overactivity; chronic alcoholism; cirrhosis; primary hyperparathyroidism; plasma-cell dyscrasia (a type of blood cell cancer); leukemia; carcinomatosis (widespread cancer metastasis); scurvy (vitamin C deficiency); chronic obstructive pulmonary disease (COPD), which is probably secondary to smoking; acromegaly; lactose intolerance. Other as yet unknown nutritional deficiencies or genetic diseases may also play a role.

It has been noted that the jaw is often involved in osteopenia and osteoporosis. Dentists have noted for years that there is an increased tooth loss with aging. This is not unexpected but what has recently been found is that the greater the loss of calcium from the spine, the greater the number of teeth lost. A fracture of the wrist is the most common fracture prior to seventy-five years of age. Though there is rarely a need for hospitalization, significant discomfort and disability do occur, often resulting in the temporary need for help with the normal activities of daily living until healing has taken place. Under these circumstances the repair process is often prolonged; and of course we can't forget the cost of additional nursing care or the mental stress of having an elderly, semi-helpless parent move in. These social and practical problems also arise if the broken bone is the shoulder (humerus).

Fractures of the spine or hip are often problematical for many years and may even contribute to the death of the victim. The frequency of collapse of the spine is unknown; however, by the age of seventy 5% of women will have had frank symptoms. Astoundingly, close to 100% of women over the age of eighty will have X-ray evidence of collapse resulting in an often significant loss of height. These fractures may occur spontaneously or after only minimal trauma such as coughing or bending and lifting. Often there are no symptoms. With the accumulation of several fractures, a round back deformity, or dowager's hump, of the mid to upper spine may become prominent, as does the obvious decrease in stature. This injury regularly leads to weeks or months of acute pain, and many years of disabling chronic back pain. The earliest suggestion that a problem may be imminent is the asymptomatic wedging seen on a routine chest or abdomen X-ray or the obvious shrinkage in height.

The femur (hip), is the site of the most devastating of

all fractures. There were 247,000 fractures in 1985 in the United States in persons over the age of forty-five; this was increased from 227,000 in 1980. Hip fracture is the most common fracture after age seventy-five and the frequency is expected to double or triple by 2050, reaching a level of approximately 650,000 people injured. This growth is due to the increasing number of the elderly, expected to reach over 20% of the population by the turn of the century. Seventy-five percent of these fractures will occur in women, half of them in the over-eighty age group. In the over-ninety population, a third of all women and a sixth of all men will break their femur.

The tragedy of all this is that these often previously productive individuals have a 12–20% greater risk of dying in the next year than individuals of the same age with other fractures. The expected risk of death is only about 9%, but it becomes progressively worse with increasing age at the time of fracture. From sixty to sixty-nine years of age, the postfracture death rate is 8.6% with an expected rate of 2%; at seventy to seventy-nine years, 13.9% (expected 5%); at eighty to eighty-nine years, 20.7% (expected 11%). Overall, 50% of persons sustaining a hip fracture will be dead in three years. So far we have just mentioned the medical aspects of this treacherous disease. In more personal terms it is known that for those who were living independently at home prior to the fracture, 15–25% will remain in a long-term nursing care facility for more than one year; and that half who are able to go home will need help and/or devices to allow them to walk and enable them to recover some portion of their independence. It has also become apparent that there is a better one-year survival rate after hospital discharge for those who are better able to ambulate. The survival rate is 93.3% if a walker is needed, 73.4% if the patient is confined in a wheelchair, and a dismal 31.5% if the patient is bedridden. Survival is also improved, the faster it takes to get surgical intervention for broken hips under way—91% if the surgery is performed in the first twenty-four hours and only 83% if undertaken after twenty-four hours.

A proper evaluation for osteoporosis should consist of a complete history and physical exam, several specific and general blood tests and an evaluation of spine and/or hip-bone density by one of several new scanning methods—qualitative X ray (QCT) or dual photon absorptiometry (DPA). The latter means is more suitable for following the effects of therapy since the amount of radiation compared to QCT is minimal.

Now let us look at the areas of prevention, education and treatment.

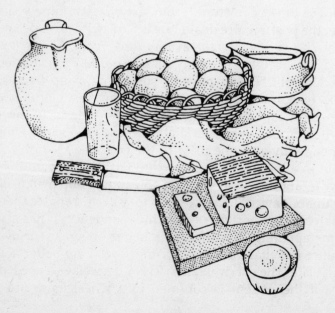

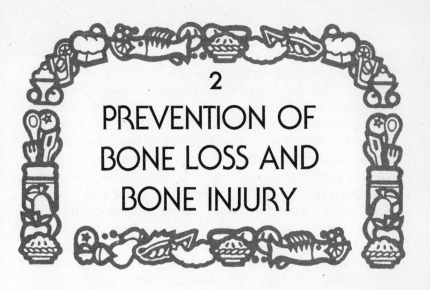

2
PREVENTION OF BONE LOSS AND BONE INJURY

Prevention is a two-pronged matter: preventing osteoporosis and preventing fracture and/or disability once osteoporosis has occurred. Prevention is the most effective treatment since, once significant osteoporosis has occurred, means of treatment other than estrogen seem to be of little or no efficacy. Therefore it is incumbent on all of us, men and women alike, to do everything possible to increase the maximal amount of bone calcium—prior to menopause in women and, even more important, prior to age thirty-five in both sexes. This can be done by maintaining an appropriate diet, exercise regimen and life-style.

Central to avoiding osteoporosis are the use of calcium and an active exercise plan. We should be taking in at least 1,000 mg of elemental calcium daily (and maybe even twice that) and do thirty minutes nonstop exercise of a moderately energetic activity at least five days out of each week.

For those individuals in jeopardy, the best prevention of injury is to injury-proof their residences. Safety training to prevent falls in the elderly is absolutely critical, since 90% of hip, forearm and pelvis fractures in the over-seventy-five age group in the United States occur from a fall. Each year almost one-third of persons over age sixty-five have a fall; and 2% of all elderly persons seek medical care for treatment of falls, a very expensive proposition indeed!

The concept of risk-proofing living spaces is really a matter of common sense: proper placement of electrical cords, removal of loose throw rugs, use of railings on stairs and rubberized bathmats, adequate lighting and, of great importance, corrective lenses. Many individuals let their vanity interfere with their common sense and neglect to wear the eyeglasses they need to see with; consequently they run into or trip over objects they cannot see. (Beware of bifocals and lenses for cataracts, which may actually impede vision.) Other considerations include the placement of cabinets in kitchens, bathrooms and other rooms, at a level that does not put the individual in a precarious balance. Chairs and beds should be at a height that allows easy access. Even shoes or slippers of an improper style or fit can cause falls. The safest footwear is the modern running shoe. Slippers should fit snugly around the entire foot and not just slip over the toes.

When an illness occurs, prolonged bed rest should be strongly discouraged; hospitalized patients should be mobilized as soon as possible. It is interesting to note that osteoporosis occurs in astronauts because of their protracted lack of weight-bearing. Another effect of illness that is often not considered, especially in the elderly, involves the side effects of medications. Recent evidence is very clear that sedative drugs such as tranquilizers, antidepressants and antipsychotics markedly increase the risk in the elderly of falling and causing bone breakage. Another commonly used group of medications that can cause problems with stability are the antihypertensives. These blood pressure–lowering drugs may be "too effective" in the aged person: they may lead to too low a blood pressure, especially when the user is standing, and may cause dizziness, fainting or "spells" and may result in falls and fractures.

Of course the most critical part of prevention is the education of the teenage girl and, even before that, her parents. Certainly males also need this, but because of the innate differences between the sexes little additional counseling needs to be done in the area of dietary calcium intake.

The two critical areas of education are exercise and diet. In both of these, females of all ages are generally deficient. The tugging on the bones during physical activity causes localized electrical currents and pressures that are immensely important in ensuring maximal bone density before age twenty-five. However, too much exercise is as bad as no exercise at all. When a woman's activity level is high and her total body fat is low, as occurs in ballet dancers, swimmers, long-distance runners, among others, her estrogen level falls and her period stops; this is very much akin to what happens during menopause. Fortunately, as recent preliminary evidence suggests, decreasing activity and/or increasing body fat will allow catch-up deposition of calcium in bones.

In our very fast-paced lives we tend to neglect proper eating; and nowhere is this truer than in the preteen and teenage female. A fast burger here, with a lunch consisting of a bag of chips; no food for three days to be able to wear the form-fitting prom dress—we all have seen this happen over and over again. One of the results is that young women get only half or less of the daily requirement of calcium, setting the invincible youth up for major traumas as a pretty vincible (as in visible and *in*visible) adult. Therefore it seems rational to supplement the diet of youths with calcium, either by convincing them of the importance of three glasses of milk a day or by adding high-calcium recipes to their diet at home. The *least* acceptable choice would be to add calcium pills to their daily intake. Supplements can be just another step toward forming the wrong attitude that taking a pill can cure or control everything. Pills may sometimes be necessary, but natural intake of calcium is certainly preferable.

Most high schools have mandatory health courses. This is the time and place to emphasize the need for exercise and proper diet. Indeed, it makes tremendous health and financial sense to start this type of education at the middle school level.

In summary, it should be obvious that prevention is the best current medicine. In lieu of that, however, for those of us, male and female, over thirty-five, the solution is to exercise safely and in moderation for 30 minutes at least five days each week and to indulge ourselves in one or more of the wonderfully exciting and bone-maintaining recipes that now await you. Go to it with vim and vigor and keep those bones strong.

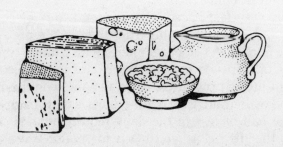

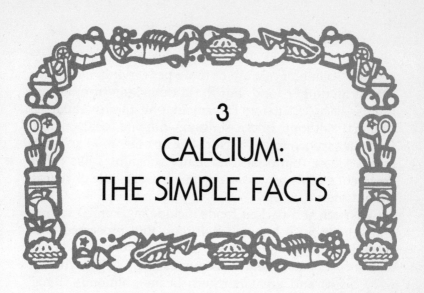

3
CALCIUM:
THE SIMPLE FACTS

"A calcium pill a day keeps the doctor away." A new twist
to an old saying reflects popular thinking about calcium
and bone health. But is that all there is to it? The flood of
recent research on this topic suggests not. In this chapter
the dietary aspects of osteoporosis will be reviewed, including calcium sources and requirements, the effects of
other nutrients on calcium utilization, and the latest news
on calcium supplementation.

CALCIUM AND THE COW

No discussion of calcium can begin without mention of
where this vital nutrient can be found. You undoubtedly
know by now that milk and other dairy products are good
sources of calcium; in fact, they are the primary suppliers

of calcium to our diet. Not only do milk, cheese and yogurt provide 300 mg of calcium or more per serving, more than almost any other food, but the combination of other nutrients—lactose, vitamin D, protein, phosphorus and magnesium, without fiber, sodium, phytate or oxalate—facilitates absorption of calcium like no other food. (Cream, cream cheese, butter and nondairy substitutes like coffee creamers and frozen desserts contain very little or no calcium, however.)

Other calcium-packed foods include mackerel, sardines and salmon with bones, smelt, and tofu processed with calcium sulfate. Moderate sources of calcium include cottage cheese, most shellfish, legumes (especially soybeans, navy beans and great northern beans), almonds, Brazil nuts, hazelnuts, bok choy, broccoli, greens (especially collard, dandelion, mustard and turnip greens) and figs. For a complete list, see the appendix at the back of the book.

HOW MUCH IS ENOUGH?

The Recommended Dietary Allowance (RDA) for calcium is currently 800 mg for children and adults, and 1,200 mg for eleven- to eighteen-year-olds and pregnant and lactating women. Recommendations have been made by numerous experts for increasing the allowance to 1,000 mg for men and premenopausal women and 1,500 mg for postmenopausal women, unless they are taking estrogen.

These allowances assume an absorption rate of calcium through the intestinal tract of about 30%, although this rate is affected by a number of factors, both nutritional and physiological. Calcium and phosphorus deficiency increase the absorption rate of calcium, but not enough to compensate for extremely low intakes. Many disease states and medications affect the absorption of calcium; some are reviewed elsewhere in this book. Epidemiologically speaking, age is probably the biggest factor for calcium utilization, however. Significantly more calcium is absorbed during high growth periods such as childhood, pregnancy and lactation, while the elderly and postmenopausal women absorb a smaller fraction of dietary calcium than do younger adults.

CALCIUM-NUTRIENT INTERACTIONS

Finally, as is the case with all nutrients, calcium absorption and use by the body depend on the form in which the calcium appears and the other foods with which it is eaten. Certain dietary components—fiber, lactose, vitamin D, caffeine and oxalic acid, to name a few—positively or negatively influence the amount of dietary calcium that can eventually be incorporated into bone. Protein and phosphorus are neutral as far as calcium utilization is concerned. The effects of sodium and some other nutrients have not clearly been established.

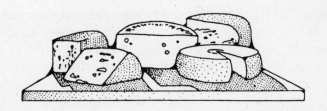

Calcium Utilization
The Effect of Dietary Components

Increase	Decrease	Neutral
lactose	fiber	phosphorus
vitamin D	phytic acid (minor)	protein
	oxalic acid	fat
	nicotine (smoking)	
	caffeine	
	excessive alcohol (long-term)	
	sodium (presumed)	

Two nutrients known to increase calcium absorption are lactose and vitamin D, both of which are found primarily in milk and milk products. This is partly why dairy foods are first-stringers in terms of calcium contribution to our diet.

Lactose, or milk sugar, is found in large amounts in milk, soft cheeses (such as cottage cheese) and ice cream. In cultured dairy products such as hard cheese and yogurt much of the lactose is converted to lactic acid by bacterial action, so the lactose content of these foods is reduced. Exactly how lactose facilitates calcium absorption is not known, but it may be related to the relatively slow rate of lactose absorption from the intestine. Glucose, a rapidly absorbed sugar, has been shown to have no effect on calcium absorption, while sorbitol actually decreases it.

Recent studies show that the calcium in dairy products is well absorbed even in those who do not digest lactose or who drink milk with lactase, the enzyme that breaks down milk sugar, added to it. This is good news for the many adults who are lactose-intolerant. Symptoms that appear after ingesting milk sugar—cramping, gas, bloating—can often be avoided by taking small amounts of milk with other foods, by using Lactaid milk or adding LactAid tablets to milk, or by getting calcium from yogurt and cheese. Knowing that the calcium in these foods will be well absorbed makes the effort worthwhile.

Vitamin D is necessary for the absorption of calcium from the intestinal tract. It is found in milk (which is fortified with the vitamin), fatty fish, cheese, butter, eggs and liver. Sunlight also transforms a vitamin D precursor to the active form in your skin. Between fifteen minutes and one hour of sun exposure a day will convert the vitamin D necessary to facilitate calcium absorption.

The production of vitamin D decreases in the elderly. Those confined indoors who also have a marginal food intake are especially prone to vitamin D deficiency. In such cases, vitamin D supplementation to the level of the RDA might be warranted. Breast milk is also low in vitamin D, and breast-fed infants are usually given supplements. In the healthy adult population, however, supplementation with vitamin D is unnecessary and may actually reduce calcium status. Excessive doses of this vitamin can damage the heart, kidney and arteries by calcification and should be avoided.

Along with calcium, fiber is certainly the "newtrient" of the eighties. Its benefits with regard to cancer, diabetes, heart disease and constipation have been proclaimed only too well in advertisements, newspapers and magazines.

In spite of all the hoopla, fiber is not the perfect food: in large amounts it does reduce the absorption of calcium. In one study, doubling the fiber intake by substituting wheat flour and bran for white flour in a typical Western diet caused the subjects to go into negative calcium balance even though their calcium intake was high. In effect, the fiber bound about 110 mg of the calcium so that it was not absorbed. In another study, increasing fiber intake with the addition of fruits and vegetables to a normal diet increased calcium intake by about 100 mg. Even so, the subjects came up short on calcium because absorption was decreased by about 300 mg per day.

Fiber, also known as bulk or roughage, is not a single nutrient, but rather the umbrella term for a number of plant components resistant to digestion by the small intestine. The exact fibrous substance that inhibits calcium uptake is not known, but cellulose, pectin and uronic acid have all been implicated.

Cellulose, found in whole-grain products such as whole-wheat bread and bran cereal, reduces calcium absorption to an unknown degree; research with pectin, found largely in fruits, has shown it to have a negligible effect. Uronic acid, present in cereals, fruits and vegetables, does bind calcium to a large extent, although most of the uronic acid in foods is broken down in the intestine, possibly releasing the calcium and making it available for absorption.

Phytic acid, a strong acid, combines with calcium and other minerals to form a salt, phytate, that cannot be absorbed. It is present in whole grains, bran, nuts and legumes. Phytate has long been held responsible for calcium imbalance and bone loss. In early-twentieth-century England, flour was supplemented with calcium carbonate as a way to reduce the incidence of rickets in children. The blame may have been misplaced, however. Phytate is broken down by bacteria and digestive enzymes in the intestine, as well as by yeast in bread and other leavened products, freeing the calcium for absorption. Evidence also exists that our bodies can adapt to a diet high in phytic acid after several weeks, resulting in an improved absorption rate for calcium. So while phytic acid does inhibit calcium absorption to some extent, its effect is probably minor, especially compared with fiber itself.

Oxalic acid is another plant substance that forms a salt (oxalate) with calcium in the intestine, presumably limiting its absorption. Since rhubarb, spinach and Swiss chard contain much more oxalic acid than calcium, it is believed that all of the calcium in these foods binds to oxalic acid and is therefore unavailable. More research needs to be done in this area, however. Whether the oxalic acid found in these vegetables and in sources such as peanuts, wheat germ and tea binds calcium from other foods eaten at the same meal is also not known. Bacteria that degrade oxalic acid have been discovered in the intestinal tract of man, leaving open the possibility that calcium might be freed for absorption.

If you had given up your beloved chocolate milk after hearing that the oxalic acid in cocoa ties up its calcium, suffer no more. The oxalate content of chocolate milk is negligible, and this drink remains an excellent source of calcium for the chocolate lover.

Does all this talk about fiber and calcium mean that you should feed your bran to the birds and ransack your pantry for the familiar cling peaches? Not yet. Moderate amounts—about 25 to 35 grams per day—eaten with a diet rich in calcium will provide you with the many benefits of fiber but won't significantly impair your calcium status. This level of fiber intake can easily be achieved with whole grains, fruits and vegetables, but you can leave the bran supplements on the supermarket shelf and occasionally enjoy plain old white bread without guilt, if you please.

Unlike fiber, the remaining factors to be reviewed that

impair calcium status—smoking, drinking caffeine, excessive alcohol and sodium use—have few, if any, redeeming qualities. Still, most of us cling to at least one of these habits and their effects on calcium deserve some discussion.

To the laundry list of dangers associated with cigarette smoking, you can add one more: an increased risk of osteoporosis. Smoking reduces estrogen levels and contributes to an early menopause, followed by accelerated bone loss. Nicotine may also directly increase calcium excretion, and its effect may be related to the alcohol and caffeine consumption that often go hand in hand with smoking.

If you are hooked on that morning cup of coffee, try adding a little milk or dry milk powder for a calcium boost. Why? It has been found that 175 mg of caffeine—the amount in 8 ounces of drip or percolated coffee—leads to a urinary calcium loss of 6 mg. This may not sound like much, but if you drink six or seven cups a day, you could lose enough calcium to make a noticeable difference in bone mass over the course of one year. Instant coffee, strong tea and some sodas also contain caffeine, roughly 30 to 90 mg per cup or can. And don't forget the caffeine in nonprescription drugs, about 200 mg per dose of weight control, diuretic and stimulant pills, and 30 to 130 mg in pain and cold medications.

Like smoking and drinking coffee, there's not much good that can be said for drinking alcohol, and its effect on calcium is no exception. Chronic alcohol abuse leads to bone demineralization, even in young adults. Alcohol directly alters the intestinal lining, so that calcium is poorly absorbed. Additionally, alcoholics frequently have impaired liver and intestinal function and eat inadequate diets, leading to deficiencies in vitamin D and calcium.

Sodium has certainly taken a backseat to other seasonings on the shelves of savvy home and restaurant chefs. A link between sodium and calcium loss may be one reason why. Several studies suggest that excessive dietary sodium leads to an increase in urinary calcium loss, although it is too early to identify the levels of sodium and calcium intake at which this becomes significant.

Phosphorus, along with calcium, is a major mineral component of bone. It is readily available in our diet and can be found in generous amounts in milk, meat, poultry and fish. The RDA for phosphorus is 800 mg per day for children and adults, and 1,200 mg for eleven- to eighteen-year-olds and pregnant and lactating women. The average daily intake in this country is between 800 and 1,200 mg, with higher intakes resulting from the heavy consumption of soft drinks, which can have up to 60 mg phosphorus per 12 ounces.

For many years, on the basis of results from animal research, excessive dietary phosphorus was thought to have a negative impact on calcium balance and bone formation. Recent studies on humans, however, have concluded that phosphorus intakes as high as 2,000 mg per day have no adverse effect on calcium metabolism. In fact, the high phosphorus diet had the beneficial effect of decreasing urinary calcium excretion without decreasing calcium absorption. The results were consistent over a range of calcium intakes between 200 and 2,000 mg per day. But the phosphoric acid in soft drinks and the forms of phosphate added to processed foods may affect calcium balance differently from the phosphorus found naturally in food.

Like phosphorus, protein has been believed to increase calcium requirements, and consumers for years have been advised to limit the consumption of meat and other high-protein foods. Recent long-term studies with high-protein diets in the form of red meat—as much as 1¼ pounds of meat taken per day—refute the earlier findings, however. The high-protein diets did not increase urinary calcium excretion, nor did they reduce the absorption of calcium or induce calcium loss. In the earlier studies, purified proteins were used, not actual dietary proteins such as meat, poultry, fish and dairy products. As previously discussed, these foods contain phosphorus, which appears to counteract the effect of the protein itself on calcium excretion.

What this means is that in terms of calcium nutrition your consumption of meat and other high-protein foods does not need to be limited. It is true, though, that as sources of saturated fat, cholesterol and calories, animal proteins should be eaten in moderate amounts, approximately 5 to 8 ounces per day for the average healthy adult.

Finally, fat has been implicated as reducing calcium absorption because fatty acids—components of dietary fat—combine with calcium in the intestine, rendering it unabsorbable. This occurs only in people with malabsorption of fat (known medically as steatorrhea) and not in healthy people. Calcium absorption has been shown to be unaffected by even relatively large amounts of dietary fat in healthy volunteers. Even so, a high-fat diet is associated with heart disease, obesity and an increased risk of some types of cancer, so a prudent diet with no more than 30% of total calories coming from fat is recommended.

As you have seen, there many dietary and related factors contributing to calcium balance and bone density. But you don't need a computer program to plan your menus; it's simpler than you might think:

1. Look to a variety of foods to meet your nutritional requirements. Relying on just a few foods—even healthy ones—can result in

nutrient imbalances, such as the effects of too much fiber and oxalate on calcium. A varied diet helps to ensure that your body will be supplied with everything it needs. Remember, you *can* get too much of a good thing!

2. As sources of calcium, phosphorus, protein, vitamin D, lactose, magnesium, manganese and other important nutrients, dairy products should not be overlooked as major players in your diet plan. Aim for at least two to three servings per day, more if you are a teenager or if you are pregnant, lactating or at risk for osteoporosis.

3. If you drink large amounts of coffee, switch to decaffeinated types, reduce your consumption, or add some milk for a calcium boost. Sodas and tea are probably best taken one hour before or several hours after high-calcium meals, to prevent possible calcium binding.

4. Give up cigarette smoking.

5. Avoid supplements of vitamin D, fiber, diuretics, diet pills, stimulants and other medication unless prescribed by your physician.

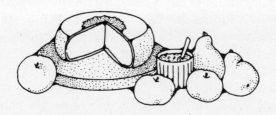

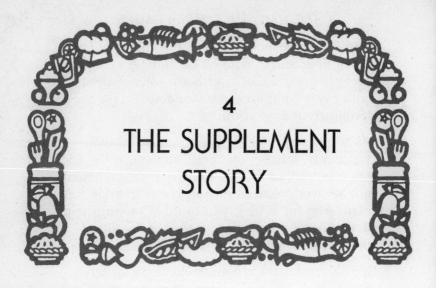

4
THE SUPPLEMENT STORY

If you're a woman and you ever watch television or read magazines, you've certainly seen the ads that so graphically depict the pained, stooped, pathetic woman you will become if you fail to take a calcium supplement. You may even believe—and understandably so—that taking calcium supplements will ensure the arrival of your golden years with good posture and a healthy glow. On the other hand, if you have an above-average interest in health and nutrition, you may have read in recent magazine and newspaper columns that taking calcium supplements will not prevent osteoporosis and in fact may not have much benefit at all. Are you thoroughly confused yet?

Calcium got the nation's attention in 1984 after the National Institutes of Health Consensus Conference on Osteoporosis. On the basis of research to date, the conference essentially concluded that the RDA for calcium should be raised from 800 mg per day for adults to 1,000 mg for men, premenopausal women and postmenopausal women on estrogen. An RDA of 1,500 mg was recommended for post-menopausal women not on estrogen, in whom calcium absorption is reduced and fracture risk is high. This started the bandwagon for supplementation, to the tune of $240 million in sales in the United States in 1986 alone.

Much research has been published in the area of calcium and bone density since then, quite a bit of it seeming to contradict earlier studies. It appears that younger women need a calcium intake of at least 1,000 mg per day to achieve calcium balance (the same amount of mineral going out of the body as coming in). But it has also been shown in several studies that a positive calcium balance—the condition that exists when more calcium is going into the body than is being excreted—for a period of two years did not result in denser bones on bone measurement tests, as would be expected. This suggests either that the calcium balance data was flawed or that calcium balance does not reflect bone density. Clearly, more research needs to be done in this area.

Likewise, it has yet to be proven that a high-calcium diet throughout life will prevent osteoporosis in later years. All we know for sure is that a deficiency of calcium will lead to bone loss. In a classic study comparing two Yugoslavian communities with similar ethnicity, level of activity and exposure to the sun but with different calcium intakes, the high-calcium group (median intake of 900 mg per day) had greater bone mass and the seniors in that group experienced half as many fractures of the leg as the seniors in the low-calcium group (median of 400 mg per day). However, the metacarpal bone densities of the two groups by the time they reached age sixty-five were nearly identical.

Some studies have shown increases in hand bone density following calcium supplementation in elderly osteoporosis patients, and others show a slowed loss of at least one type of bone, after calcium supplementation of 800 to 1,000 mg per day for postmenopausal women.

Still other researchers had quite different results. Riis and others at the University of Copenhagen compared bone densities for several body sites over a two-year period in forty-three women in their early postmenopausal years. Those taking 2,000 mg calcium daily had a slightly slowed loss of dense bone in the body compared with women taking a placebo, but bone losses from the spine and parts of the forearm were similar. Only women in the estrogen-treated group retained their bone mass. In other words, even the large doses of calcium taken did little to arrest bone loss in this population. It appears, however, that 1,500 mg calcium taken daily along with .3 mg estrogen—half the usual dose—does slow postmenopausal bone loss or even increase bone mass of the spongy trabecular bone.

What does all this mean? Part of the confusion stems from the fact that the researchers measured various types of bones and tested bone densities at different postmenopausal ages. Trying to compare the data from two studies, then, may be like comparing *The Wall Street Journal* and *Better Homes and Gardens:* both are valid sources but each gives you completely different information.

In the studies that have been done, two different types of bone have been measured: dense cortical bone and spongy trabecular bone. If the hand or upper part of the forearm is tested for bone loss, cortical bone is measured. When the spine, wrist or part of the forearm near the wrist is tested, primarily trabecular bone is measured. The two types of bones differ in composition and in rate of loss. Cortical bone is lost at a rapid rate just after menopause, while spongy bone is lost at a steady rate after age thirty. Calcium affects the loss of dense bone, but not the softer bone of the wrist and spine; therefore, results of a research study depend on where the bone is measured, and at what point in menopause the tests are conducted. If cortical bone is measured, especially if it is just before menopause or after age seventy, the effect of calcium supplementation on bone density will be much more favorable than if spongy bone is measured during the immediate postmenopausal years.

This all boils down to the following:

- Calcium supplementation cannot be said to prevent osteoporosis, especially if it is delayed until menopausal years.

- Adequate calcium intake (approximately 1,000 mg per day) throughout life will at least reduce the risk of fracture of dense bone, such as the leg, hip, hand and upper forearm bones.

- The effectiveness of calcium supplementation in postmenopausal women is greatly increased by the addition of small amounts of estrogen.

So you know that you need to get enough calcium in your diet: between 1,000 and 1,500 mg per day, depending on your stage in life. You know that popping calcium pills is not a panacea for osteoporosis. You even know that other foods and substances that you ingest will affect your calcium balance and bone integrity. So now what do you do?

First, take a good look at your current diet. It might be helpful to write down everything that you eat for three to five days, including Saturday and/or Sunday. Count how many high-calcium foods you eat per day. High calcium sources are those providing about 300 mg calcium in one serving. A cup of milk or yogurt, 1½ ounces of hard cheese (not cottage cheese) and 1 cup of pudding all qualify, as do 3 ounces of sardines, ½ cup of tofu, 3 stalks of fresh broccoli and 1 cup of cooked collard greens.

How many high-calcium servings would you have gotten if this had been your menu for one day?

	MENU	HIGH CALCIUM SOURCES
Breakfast:	½ cup milk	½
	1 cup corn flakes	
	6 ounces orange juice	
Lunch:	Chef salad with cheese and blue cheese dressing	1 or more
	roll with butter	
	diet soda	
Snack:	apple	
Dinner:	3 ounces baked chicken	½
	1 baked potato with sour cream	
	1 cup broccoli, frozen	
	½ cup pudding	
	hot tea	
Snack:	½ cup cottage cheese	
	¼ cup raisins	

You would have eaten the equivalent of two high calcium sources, providing about 600 mg calcium. The next step is to identify other calcium sources in your diet. Refer to the appendix, "Food Sources of Calcium," pages 160–166, for assistance. For the sample day, other calcium sources include the cup of broccoli at dinner and the ½ cup of cottage cheese in the evening, for about 125 mg added calcium. Although broccoli can be a major source of calcium, the portion in the sample menu was small and came from frozen, so it contributed only about 50 mg to the day's total.

You don't actually need to add up the exact calcium contribution from these medium sources, but rather get a general idea of whether or not it is significant. If you regularly eat foods that contain some calcium, like shrimp salad, refried beans, cream soup and frozen yogurt, for example, your calcium total could be raised by 300 mg or more per day. If most of these foods are only occasionally or never eaten, however, the daily calcium contribution would average under 100 mg.

Once you've estimated the calcium in your diet from high and medium food sources, you can add 50 to 100 mg to account for the small amount of calcium from the remaining foods in your diet. Then compare this total to your calcium requirement. (Remember, at least 1,000 mg is thought necessary for healthy adults, with 1,200 mg required for teenagers and pregnant and lactating women.) In the sample menu above, about 800 mg of calcium was eaten from all sources.

Shortfalls in your calcium intake should first be corrected by improving your diet. This is preferable to popping calcium pills because other nutrients in the food you eat will facilitate calcium utilization. Additionally, calcium in supplement form may inhibit the absorption of other essential nutrients like manganese, and at least a few experts are concerned about possible long-term side effects from large doses of the substances that carry the calcium in supplements.

The ways to increase the calcium in your diet are limited only by your imagination and sense of adventure. Can you make a point of drinking milk with your muffin in the morning, or adding a quick breakfast shake if you usually run out with nothing in your stomach? The calorie content is a poor excuse for not drinking milk; nonfat milk has only 80 calories per glass—less than the amount in one average cookie—and the calories are well spent. If you don't like it plain, try flavoring your milk with chocolate. Look for sugar-free brands at the supermarket to avoid the extra calories, if desired.

Cheese makes a high-calcium substitute for meat in sandwiches, with one of the low-fat varieties a good choice if fat or calories are a concern. Feta and hoop cheeses are tasty additions to tossed salads, as are tofu, anchovies and chickpeas (garbanzo beans). All are good calcium sources. Many other ideas can be found in the recipe section of this book and on the Top Ten Tips list, pages 46–47.

How can the calcium in the sample menu be increased? Adding another ½ cup of milk at breakfast, substituting sour cream with seasoned plain yogurt on the potato and having figs instead of raisins with the cottage cheese snack would bring the calcium total over 1,000 mg without increasing the calories. So would switching the cottage cheese to 1 ounce of cheddar cheese and adding more broccoli or another vegetable, such as a romaine lettuce salad, at dinner.

Advertisers have not let us go without noticing all the new calcium-fortified foods on the market—cereal, flour, soda and many others. But are they worthwhile?

Well . . . maybe. The extra calcium won't hurt, but whether it will be absorbed is another question that as yet has no definitive answer. If the form of added calcium is calcium triphosphate, an insoluble salt, the benefits are probably minimal. The phosphoric acid in sodas may also make the added calcium unavailable. So before you buy, check the label, and at least for now don't rely on these foods as your major sources of dietary calcium.

After you develop some strategies for getting more calcium in your diet, again compare your calcium intake to the recommended level. If your intake still falls short, you can make up the difference with a calcium supplement.

People who can't drink milk often question me about taking a calcium supplement. Even if you are lactose-intolerant, supplementation is not the immediate solution; you *can* get adequate amounts of calcium in your diet. Lactose—milk sugar—is usually broken down by an enzyme called lactase into two smaller sugars, glucose and galactose, which are then absorbed. Lactose-intolerants have insufficient amounts of lactase, so bacteria in the intestines act on the milk sugar, forming lactic acid and gases, which lead to a bloated feeling, gas, cramping and diarrhea. Many people with lactose intolerance can drink small amounts of milk with meals, however, without the unpleasant symptoms. Others use Lactaid milk or add LactAid, lactase in tablet form, to their milk. Such preparations break down the lactose without affecting the milk's calcium content. Since most of the lactose is broken down to lactic acid in cultured dairy products such as buttermilk, hard cheese, yogurt and frozen yogurt, these foods are usually well tolerated—contrary to popular opinion—except in the most severe cases.

If you are lactose-intolerant, try taking smaller amounts

of the lactose-containing foods—milk, cottage cheese and other soft cheeses, ice cream—as part of your meal. Rely on cultured dairy products and other high-calcium foods like tofu, broccoli and salmon to boost your calcium intake. Many of the recipes in this book, like the Tofu Shake and Salmon-Tofu Patties, are made without dairy products.

Many questions come to mind when calcium supplementation is considered. How much to take? What kind? When during the day? First, supplements are meant to do just what they say—*supplement* your diet, not replace foods in it. The amount that you need to take depends on how much calcium you're getting from the food you eat, as well as other factors. For example, kidney-stone formers should probably not take supplements at all because the calcium is not conserved normally and will end up in the urine, increasing the risk for calcium oxalate stone formation. (There is no conclusive evidence to support a low-calcium diet, however, and it may lead to bone loss. Kidney stones are probably most effectively treated with medication rather than by diet.) The maximum amount that *anyone* would need to supplement is 1,500 mg of calcium per day, but your needs are probably much lower, if any at all.

When deciding which supplement would be most appropriate for you, look at the milligram amount of elemental calcium rather than the tablet size. If you are going to be taking a large dose, the calcium will be better utilized and probably better tolerated if you divide the dose and take two or three smaller pills throughout the day rather than one large one.

There are many acceptable supplements available on the market. Calcium carbonate has the highest percentage of elemental calcium—40%—so fewer pills are needed compared with other forms. It is also the least expensive form of supplement, especially the generic products.

When you swallow a tablet, it must disintegrate and then dissolve in your stomach before the calcium can be absorbed. Chewing a supplement increases its surface area and may enhance the absorption. Calcium carbonate needs an acid environment to dissolve, and many brands do not

Acceptable Calcium Supplements

NAME	FORM	PERCENT OF CALCIUM IN CALCIUM COMPLEX	TABLET SIZE (mg)	ELEMENTAL CALCIUM PER TABLET (mg)
Alka-Mints	carbonate	40	850	340
Alka-2	carbonate	40	500	200
Calcitrel	carbonate	40	N/A	234
Cal-Sup	carbonate	40	750	300
Caltrate 600	carbonate	40	1,500	600
Centrum*	phosphate	29	N/A	162
Lilly	gluconate	9	486	44
Lilly	lactate	13	648	84
One-A-Day maximum formula*	carbonate	40	N/A	130
Os-Cal 500 tablets	carbonate	40	1250	500
Oyster Shell Calcium	carbonate	40	500	200
Titralac	carbonate	40	420	168
Tums	carbonate	40	500	200
Tums E-X	carbonate	40	750	300
Within*	carbonate	40	N/A	300

*multivitamin-mineral preparation
**multivitamin preparation with iron

dissolve well, especially in older people and others with decreased gastric acidity. If you have achlorhydria—impaired gastric acid secretion—take your supplement with meals. The food itself will generate enough acid to break down the calcium carbonate. The supplement chart that follows includes calcium carbonate products that will be at least 75% dissolved within thirty minutes after being swallowed. Supplements in liquid form are also available.

Some manufacturers claim that it is better to take your calcium with added vitamin A and/or vitamin D. Since both A and D can be toxic in large doses and because evidence shows that calcium is better utilized if taken alone, leave those preparations on the store shelf. Vitamins A and D are readily available in foods and multivitamin preparations, and the sun converts vitamin D in our skin to the active form. Likewise, there is no evidence for taking other minerals, such as magnesium, with your calcium supplement. Two calcium preparations—dolomite and bone meal—should be avoided because of possible lead contamination. Oyster-shell calcium, on the other hand, is calcium carbonate and is perfectly safe.

Calcium tablets are generally best taken between meals, to avoid possible interaction with other food substances or nutrients. Some experts suggest taking your supplement before bedtime, to suppress calcium removal from bone at night. This theory has yet to be tested, however. If you develop stomach pain, gas, bloating or other symptoms after ingesting the supplement, try taking it with meals, preferably dairy products. The other food should alleviate or reduce the symptoms, and the vitamin D and lactose in milk products will facilitate absorption of the calcium. Taking the supplement in smaller doses may also be beneficial.

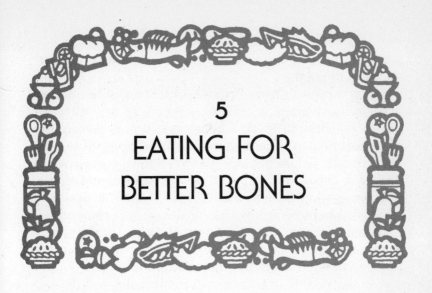

5
EATING FOR BETTER BONES

There is much yet to be discovered about calcium, bone health and osteoporosis prevention. But not having all the answers should not prevent you from practicing what will increase your chances of having strong, healthy bones throughout life. Most of the dietary recommendations in this book have numerous other health benefits. The very fact that the many reasons and ways to stay healthy and fit reinforce each other tends to verify their validity. To summarize what has been covered in detail already and what you can do for better bones:

• Enjoy a variety of foods, including dairy products and other high calcium sources. Don't go overboard with fiber, or with those foods high in oxalic acid—spinach, rhubarb and Swiss chard. Moderation regarding sodium, alcohol and caffeine consumption is a good idea. Quit smoking.

• Avoid unnecessary supplementation with vitamin A, vitamin D, calcium, fiber and other vitamin-mineral preparations and over-the-counter drugs. They usually do more harm than good.

• If you can't squeeze in at least 1,000 mg of calcium per day on the average, a calcium supplement can bring you up to the desired level. Choose one that is readily dissolvable and convenient and of the appropriate dosage for your needs. Before bedtime, between meals or when eating dairy foods are the best times for supplementation. If you are getting close to the RDA for calcium in your diet and are otherwise at low risk for developing osteoporosis (you have a large bone structure; are active, healthy, non-Caucasian; have no family history; and so on), supplementation is probably not indicated.

• Walk, run, play tennis, racketball, volleyball, basketball, whatever: exercise! Activities that put weight on your muscles and bones through the force of gravity are best, but all forms of exercise are beneficial.

• When you reach menopause, discuss with your doctor the pros and cons of estrogen supplementation in your particular situation. There are many factors involved in deciding to take estrogen or not, but taking it is the most effective way at present to arrest postmenopausal bone loss.

Top Ten Tips for Boosting Your Bone Calcium

1. Add ⅓ cup to ½ cup nonfat dry milk to recipes for pancakes, breads, mashed potatoes, scrambled eggs, pudding, cookies, cakes and other foods. The milk powder can be blended into the other dry ingredients (flour, sugar, etc.) or added along with the water or liquid milk.

2. Substitute yogurt for sour cream in beef Stroganoff, gelatin desserts, dips, dressings and toppings.

3. Choose spinach, romaine and other brightly colored salad greens instead of iceberg lettuce.

4. Use milk or buttermilk instead of water to reconstitute canned soups, dry cereal such as Cream of Wheat, instant mashed potatoes and salad dressing mixes.

5. When feeding your sweet tooth, think calcium as well as calories. Pudding, frozen yogurt, ice milk and custard pack lots of nutritional bang for the calorie buck.

6. Double-strength milk is now appearing in grocery dairy cases; however, you can make your own more cheaply by adding nonfat dry milk powder to the regular milk you buy. Blending in ⅓ cup dry milk per 1 cup liquid milk will double the calcium content and make the milk richer without altering the taste.

7. Substitute half the mayonnaise in salad dressings and dips with plain yogurt. Dry soup or dressing mix can be added to liven up the flavor, if desired.

8. Lighten your coffee by adding milk or evaporated milk instead of cream. Or, for convenience, use nonfat dry milk powder rather than nondairy creamer. *Cream and cream substitutes are loaded with fat and calories but are poor calcium sources.*

9. Mix lemon juice, a few drops of olive oil, crushed garlic and grated Parmesan cheese for a low-calorie, high-calcium salad dressing.

10. Top casseroles, omelettes, toast, baked potatoes and steamed vegetables with shredded cheddar, Swiss or mozzarella cheese for a tasty calcium boost.

MENU SUGGESTIONS FOR THE CALCIUM-CONSCIOUS DINER

There are many restaurant menu items that are high in calcium; a few suggestions are listed below. To reduce the calorie count, use as little dressing, butter, sour cream and cream sauce as possible. Seafood dishes are especially lean.

Appetizers
artichoke with lemon
crab cocktail
cream soups
French onion soup
fried cheese sticks
nachos with cheese
oysters on the half shell
potato skins with cheese
seafood or shrimp salad
shrimp cocktail
steamed clams

Beverages
Kahlúa and milk
low-fat or nonfat milk
milk shake

Continental dishes
cheese crêpe
cheese omelette
chef salad
chicken Cordon Bleu
chili and cornbread
cobb salad
peasant lunch (cheese cubes, fresh fruit, bread)

quiche
salad with dark greens, fresh vegetables, cheeses and
    chickpeas (garbanzo beans) or kidney beans
sandwiches made with cheese or meat and cheese
steamed vegetable plate with cheese sauce

Eastern dishes
bean curd (tofu) dishes
beef with broccoli
sautéed broccoli or bok choy
scallops with bean curd
shrimp with black bean sauce
shrimp with snow peas
sweet-and-sour shrimp
other shrimp, scallop and lobster dishes

Italian dishes
antipasto salad
Caesar salad
cheese pizza with anchovies
eggplant parmigiana
lasagne
linguine with white clam sauce
tortellini stuffed with ricotta cheese
veal parmigiana
other meat and cheese or pasta and
    cheese combinations

Mexican dishes
bean burritos
chiles rellenos
enchiladas
flautas
huevos rancheros
quesadillas
other cheese or bean dishes

Seafood dishes
bouillabaise
coquilles St.-Jacques
king crab
linguine with clam sauce
lobster tail
shrimp scampi
sole meunière
other shellfish dishes

A NOTE ON THE RECIPES

The 100 recipes in this book were designed with both your health and your palate in mind. They are, of course, rich in calcium from a variety of food sources, including dairy products, legumes, seafood, vegetables, fruits and nuts.

But they also follow current recommendations for the American diet. They are low in fat, moderate to high in fiber and complex carbohydrates and prudent in protein and sugar content. As an added benefit, the relatively low fat and sugar content of the recipes translates into dishes that are low in calories, especially compared to traditional recipes.

Since most modern cooks cannot afford to spend all day in the kitchen, the recipes were written to be as quick and convenient as possible without compromising taste, appeal or nutritional value.

PART II

Recipes

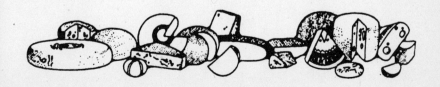

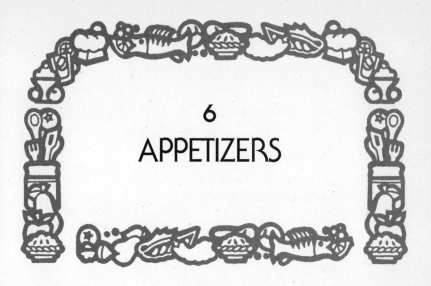

6
APPETIZERS

TOASTED FISH CANAPÉS

Number of servings: 6

>   1 3½-ounce can sardines, packed in oil
>   ¼ teaspoon Worcestershire sauce
>   1 tablespoon finely minced onion
>   1 tablespoon finely chopped parsley
>   2 tablespoons diet mayonnaise
>   6 thin slices soft bread, white or wheat

Drain and mash sardines. Mix with Worcestershire sauce, onion, parsley and mayonnaise. Cut the crusts from the slices of bread. Spread the sardine mixture on the bread. Roll the slices and secure them with toothpicks. Toast immediately before serving, if desired.

Calories per serving: 100
Calcium per serving: 102 mg

LITE AND LEAN NACHOS

Special preparation methods result in nachos exceptionally low in fat but high in flavor.

Number of Servings: 4

> **6 6-inch corn tortillas**
> **vegetable oil spray**
> **salt**
> **1 15-ounce can pinto beans, drained**
> **3 ounces (³/₄ cup) shredded cheddar cheese**
> **2 small tomatoes, chopped**
> **2 green onions, chopped**
> **¼ cup plain yogurt**

Cut each tortilla into 6 wedges, like a pie. Spread wedges in a single layer on cookie sheet. Spray with vegetable oil spray and sprinkle with salt. Bake at 375 degrees for about 5 minutes. Turn wedges over and sprinkle with salt. Bake for about 5 more minutes or until crispy. Mash pinto beans with a potato masher or fork, and heat thoroughly over medium heat, stirring occasionally. Spread tortilla chips on a heatproof platter; top with beans and cheese. Bake at 375 degrees for about 5 minutes, until cheese melts. Top with tomatoes, onions and yogurt.

Calories per serving: 288
Calcium per serving: 282 mg

SALTED PRAWNS

Delicious with a colorful tray of raw vegetables.

Number of servings: 6

> **1 pound unshelled medium shrimp**
> **2 tablespoons cornstarch**
> **1–1½ cups vegetable oil (enough almost to cover**
>   **shrimp)**
> **1 teaspoon salt**

Cut legs from shrimp but do not remove shells. Rinse shrimp thoroughly, drain and allow to dry in colander for about 15 minutes. Place shrimp in bowl; add cornstarch and mix to coat shrimp. Heat oil in wok until very hot. Add shrimp and fry about 1 minute (until shrimp just turns opaque). Drain shrimp on paper towel and remove oil from wok. A light film of oil will remain. Over high flame reheat wok; add shrimp, then salt. Cook and stir for 45 seconds. Turn onto heated platter and serve immediately.

Calories per serving: 134
Calcium per serving: 48 mg

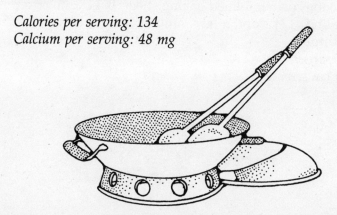

SEASONED MOZZARELLA SNACKS

Number of servings: 12 2-piece servings

8 ounces part-skim mozzarella cheese
2 eggs
1 tablespoon nonfat milk
¾ cup dry bread crumbs
2 teaspoons Italian seasoning, crushed
2 teaspoons garlic powder
1½ tablespoons chopped parsley
¼ cup unsifted flour

Cut cheese into 24 1-inch square cubes; set aside. In a pie pan beat eggs and milk. In another pie pan combine bread crumbs, Italian seasoning, garlic powder and chopped parsley. Place flour in a small bowl. Coat cheese cubes completely with flour, then egg mixture, and finally with bread crumbs. Repeat egg and bread-crumb coatings. Place in a single layer on a plate, cover with foil, and refrigerate 2–3 hours or overnight. Preheat oven to 400 degrees. Place cheese cubes on a foil-lined baking sheet. Bake until crisp, 6–7 minutes. Let stand a few minutes before serving.

Calories per serving: 82 for 2 pieces
Calcium per serving: 149 mg for 2 pieces

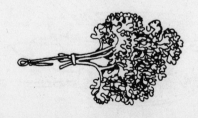

STUFFED BREAD ROLLS

Number of servings: 24 slices

> **1 16-ounce loaf frozen bread dough**
> **1 bunch Swiss chard**
> **3 ounces (¾ cup) shredded cheddar cheese**
> **1 egg, beaten**
> **2 tablespoons minced onion**
> **1 tablespoon margarine**
> **½ teaspoon garlic powder**
> **2 tablespoons grated Parmesan cheese**

Let bread dough thaw to room temperature according to package directions. Boil Swiss chard 15–20 minutes in covered pot with 1–2 inches water. Drain well and cool. Mix Swiss chard, cheddar cheese, egg and onion. Cut dough in half. On lightly floured board, roll out dough into two 8×10-inch rectangles. Spread Swiss chard mixture over dough to within 1 inch of edges. Beginning with long side, roll up tightly. Lightly grease or spray bottom of a 9×13-inch pan. Place dough rolls in pan, seam down. Melt margarine and combine with garlic powder and Parmesan cheese; brush on top of rolls. Let rolls rise until tripled. Bake at 375 degrees for 25–30 minutes or until golden brown. Cut each roll into 12 slices.

Calories per serving: 154 for 2 slices
Calcium per serving: 112 mg for 2 slices

CLASSIC ARTICHOKE

The artichoke is simpler to prepare than you might think.

Number of servings: 4

> **2 large artichokes**
> **4–5 quarts water**
> **1 tablespoon olive oil**
> **1½ tablespoons lemon juice**
> **1 clove garlic, cut into fourths**
> **½ teaspoon salt**

Remove any discolored leaves and the small leaves at the base of each artichoke. Trim stem to be even with the base. Cut 1 inch off the top of each artichoke and snip off points of leaves. Rinse artichokes. In a large kettle heat water, oil, lemon juice, garlic and salt to boiling. Add artichokes. Heat to boiling; reduce heat. Simmer, uncovered, rotating occasionally, until leaves pull out easily, about 30–40 minutes. Using tongs, remove artichokes carefully from water. Place upside down to drain. Serve with diet mayonnaise or Light Italian Dip, page 130.

Calories per serving: 33
Calcium per serving: 26 mg

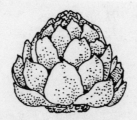

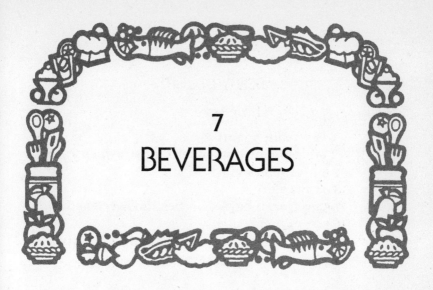

7

BEVERAGES

TROPICAL TEASER

Number of servings: 3

> 1 cup pineapple juice
> ½ cup evaporated nonfat milk
> ⅓ cup instant nonfat dry milk
> ¼ teaspoon coconut extract or to taste
> ½ teaspoon rum extract or to taste
> 1 ripe medium banana, sliced
> 6 ice cubes

Pour pineapple juice and evaporated milk into a blender, add dry milk and blend until smooth. Add extracts and sliced banana and blend again until smooth. Add ice cubes, one at a time, and blend on low speed after each one, until smooth. Blend on high until thick and frothy, about 30 seconds.

Calories per serving: 129
Calcium per serving: 220 mg

BERRY DELIGHT

Number of servings: 2 1-cup servings

> **1 cup plain yogurt**
> **2 tablespoons boysenberry or strawberry jam**
>   **or preserves**
> **1 cup water**
> **¾ cup frozen boysenberries, unsweetened**

Blend ingredients in a blender until smooth, adding berries slowly.

Calories per serving: 151
Calcium per serving: 225 mg

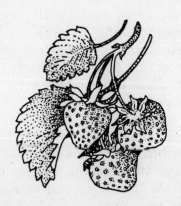

MOCHA INSTANT BREAKFAST

. . . with just enough caffeine to get you going in the morning!

Number of servings: 2

> ¾ **cup whole milk, very cold**
> ⅔ **cup instant nonfat dry milk**
> ½ **teaspoon instant coffee**
> 2 **teaspoons cocoa**
> 1 **tablespoon sugar**
> **pinch of salt**
> 5 **ice cubes**

Blend liquid milk and dry milk in blender. Add coffee, cocoa, sugar and salt and blend until smooth. Add ice cubes, one at a time, and blend on low speed after each one, until smooth. Blend on high for 30 seconds, until thick and frothy.

Calories per serving: 163
Calcium per serving: 391 mg

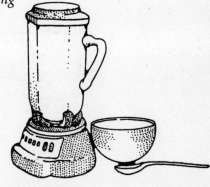

OLD-FASHIONED HOT COCOA

Number of servings: 6 1-cup servings

> **5 tablespoons sugar**
> **⅓ cup cocoa**
> **¼ teaspoon salt**
> **1½ cups water**
> **4½ cups whole milk**
> **1 cup instant nonfat dry milk**
> **½ teaspoon mint extract (optional)**

Mix sugar, cocoa and salt in a 2-quart saucepan. Add water. Heat to boiling, stirring constantly. Boil and stir for 2 minutes. Stir in liquid milk and then slowly add dry milk, stirring continuously. Heat thoroughly but do not boil. Stir in extract, if desired. Just before serving, beat with a hand beater until foamy.

Calories per serving: 202
Calcium per serving: 365 mg

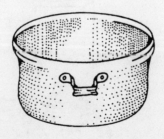

TOFU SHAKE

Tofu, a versatile protein and calcium source, is the basis for this quick breakfast drink.

Number of servings: 6 1-cup servings

> **3 cups orange juice**
> **1 14-ounce package soft tofu**
> **2 ripe bananas**

Blend orange juice and tofu in blender. Slice in banana and blend until smooth.

Calories per serving: 138
Calcium per serving: 97 mg

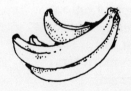

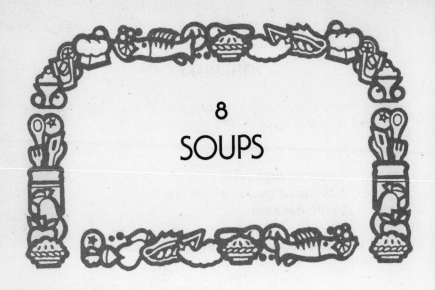

8
SOUPS

BOSTON-STYLE CLAM CHOWDER

Number of servings: 6 ³/₄-cup servings

 1½ cups chicken broth
 2 cups diced cauliflower
 1 cup peeled and cubed potato
 1 cup chopped onion
 1 cup sliced mushrooms
 1 teaspoon dill weed
 ¼ teaspoon marjoram
 ½ teaspoon salt
     dash pepper
 1 cup evaporated nonfat milk
 1 10-ounce can clams, drained
     chopped parsley

Heat broth to boiling and add cauliflower. Cover and heat to boiling; simmer 10–12 minutes. With a strainer, remove cauliflower and let cool. To broth add potato, onion, mushrooms, dill weed, marjoram, salt and pepper, and return to a boil. Cover and simmer 15 minutes, stirring occasionally. While soup is cooking, blend cauliflower and milk in a blender until smooth. After soup has cooked for 15 minutes, gradually add pureed cauliflower to soup, stirring over low heat until thick. Add clams. Turn up to medium heat and bring to a boil. Boil 1 minute. Pour into soup bowls and garnish with parsley.

Calories per serving: 103
Calcium per serving: 167 mg

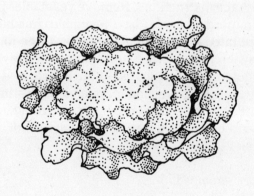

CREAM OF BROCCOLI SOUP

Number of servings: 5 ³/₄-cup servings

  2 cups chicken broth
  1 10-ounce package frozen chopped broccoli
  4 tablespoons chopped parsley
  1 medium onion, chopped
  2 tablespoons lemon juice
  2 cups evaporated nonfat milk
  1 tablespoon cornstarch
    dash nutmeg
  2 teaspoons garlic salt
  ¹/₈ teaspoon pepper
    parsley

Heat broth with broccoli, parsley, onion and lemon juice to boiling. Cover and heat until broccoli is tender, according to package instructions. Remove vegetables from broth with a strainer and cool. Place vegetables in a blender and add evaporated milk until blender is three-fourths full. Add cornstarch and blend until smooth. Slowly stir the broccoli-milk mixture, the rest of the evaporated milk, and the nutmeg, garlic salt and pepper into the broth. Heat over low flame until thickened, stirring constantly. Bring to a boil and boil lightly for 1 minute. Serve hot, garnished with parsley.

Calories per serving: 125
Calcium per serving: 355 mg

CREAM OF MUSHROOM SOUP

It's actually milk, not cream, that makes this soup light, lively, and rich in calcium.

Number of servings: 6 ⅔-cup servings

> 8 ounces fresh mushrooms
> 1 cup chopped onion
> 2 tablespoons margarine
> 1 teaspoon salt
> ⅛ teaspoon white pepper
> 2 cups chicken broth (if bouillon or salted broth is used, omit 1 teaspoon salt)
> 3 tablespoons cornstarch
> 1 12-ounce can evaporated nonfat milk
> snipped parsley

Slice enough mushrooms to measure 1 cup; chop remaining mushrooms. Cook and stir sliced mushrooms in nonstick skillet over low heat until golden. Set aside. In medium-size saucepan, cook and stir chopped mushrooms and onion in margarine until onion is tender; stir in salt and pepper. Cook and stir over low heat, about 1 minute. Remove from heat. Stir in chicken broth. Heat to boiling, stirring occasionally. Blend cornstarch into milk until smooth. Stir milk and sliced mushrooms into broth. Bring to boil; boil 1 minute. Remove from heat. Serve garnished with parsley.

Calories per serving: 127
Calcium per serving: 198 mg

CREAM OF SPINACH SOUP

A thick, spicy soup packed with nutrition.

Number of servings: 6 ⅔-cup servings

> 1 10-ounce package frozen chopped spinach (or
>   1½ cups fresh cooked spinach)
> ½ cup nonfat dry milk
> 3 cups nonfat milk
> 2 tablespoons minced white onion
> 1 tablespoon cornstarch
> 1 teaspoon salt
> ½ teaspoon pepper
> ¼–½ teaspoon curry

Cook frozen spinach according to package instructions. Drain and let cool. Blend nonfat dry milk with liquid milk until smooth and free of lumps. Run spinach and onion through a food processor or blender until smooth. (The mixture doesn't need to be completely pureed.) Add cornstarch to ½ cup of the milk mixture in a small container, cover and shake to blend. Combine milk, cornstarch mixture, salt, pepper, curry and spinach mixture in a saucepan and heat over low flame until thickened, stirring constantly. Increase flame and heat to boiling. Remove from heat and serve.

Calories per serving: 88
Calcium per serving: 305 mg

CREAMY RICE SOUP

A delicious change-of-pace soup.

Number of servings: 8 ³/₄-cup servings

> **1 cup diced cauliflower**
> **2 cups chicken or beef broth**
> **2 cups nonfat milk**
> **²/₃ cup nonfat dry milk**
> **1¹/₂ cups cooked rice**
> **1 teaspoon salt**
> **3 green onions, sliced diagonally**
> **2 egg yolks, beaten well**

Cook cauliflower in broth until tender, 10–12 minutes. Remove from broth with strainer and cool slightly. Place cooked cauliflower, liquid milk and dry milk in blender and blend until smooth. Add milk mixture, rice, salt and green onions to broth and heat over low flame, stirring constantly, until hot and at desired consistency. Just before serving, stir in beaten egg yolks, letting them drop through a fine strainer into hot soup.

Calories per serving: 117
Calcium per serving: 176 mg

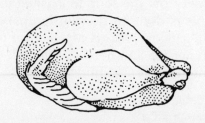

HEARTY BEAN SOUP

Serve with a green salad and cornbread.

Number of servings: 12 main-dish servings

> 1 pound navy beans, washed and drained
> 3 quarts water
> 2 smoked ham hocks
> 1 10¾-ounce can beef broth
> 2 cloves garlic, minced
> 1 bay leaf
> ½ teaspoon salt
> ½ teaspoon pepper
> 2 cups mashed potato
> 3 medium onions, chopped
> 1½ cups diced celery, with leaves
> ¼ cup finely chopped parsley
> 2 cups diced carrot
> 2 tablespoons cider vinegar

Cover dry beans with water in a soup pot, bring to a boil and boil 2 minutes. Remove from heat, cover and allow to stand for 1 hour. After 1 hour, add ham hocks, beef broth, garlic, bay leaf, salt and pepper to the beans. Simmer, covered, for 2 hours. Remove ham hocks; trim fat and bone from ham and cut ham into pieces and set aside. Add a little liquid from the soup to mashed potato to thin until runny (this is done to prevent lumps). Stir potato, onions, celery, parsley, carrots and ham into the soup. Cover and simmer for another 1–1½ hours. Stir in cider vinegar. Let simmer a few minutes more.

Calories per serving: 200
Calcium per serving: 78 mg

MARVELOUS MEATLESS CHILI

Great for leftovers, this low-calorie chili is one of Judy's favorites.

Number of servings: 16 ³/₄-cup servings

- 1½ cups sliced carrot
- 1½ cups chopped onion
- 1½ cups chopped green pepper
- 1½ cups sliced celery
- 1 15-ounce can stewed tomatoes
- 1 15-ounce can tomato puree (or tomato sauce)
- 1 6-ounce can tomato paste
- 1 6-ounce can tomato juice
  juice of 1 lemon
- 2 15-ounce cans kidney beans, drained (reserve liquid)
- 1 15-ounce can chickpeas (garbanzo beans), drained
- 3 medium cloves garlic, minced
- 2–3 tablespoons chili powder
- 1 teaspoon sugar
- 1½ teaspoons dried basil
- 1 teaspoon salt
- ½ teaspoon pepper
- ½ teaspoon red pepper sauce

Heat cut-up vegetables in a large nonstick pot until just barely tender, stirring occasionally. Add rest of ingredients and mix well. If too thick, add reserved kidney bean juice. Cover and simmer for about 20 minutes. Do not overcook or vegetables will be mushy.

Calories per serving: 122
Calcium per serving: 48 mg

MUSTARD GREEN SOUP

Number of servings: 10 ³/₄-cup servings

> **1 small bundle mustard greens**
> **8 cups chicken stock**
> **1 tablespoon fish sauce**
> **½ tablespoon sugar**
> **2 green onions, chopped**
> **3–4 thin slices fresh ginger**

Remove root ends and imperfect leaves from mustard greens. Wash greens thoroughly and drain. Heat stock; add all ingredients except mustard greens and simmer for 10 minutes. Add mustard greens and simmer 3 more minutes. Serve hot.

Calories per serving: 39
Calcium per serving: 34 mg

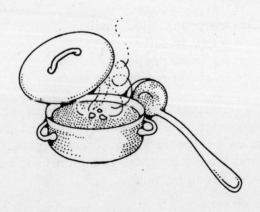

TOFU CHICKEN SOUP

Number of servings: 8 1-cup servings

> **4 cups broth (chicken stock or canned chicken broth)**
> **3 cups chopped Chinese cabbage**
> **2 stalks celery (about ½ cup)**
> **1 cup sliced mushrooms**
> **2 cups cubed tofu (about 11 ounces)**
> **1 cup shredded, cooked skinless chicken breast**
> **few drops sesame oil**
> **2 green onions, finely chopped**

Bring broth to boil in saucepan. Add cabbage, cover and simmer for about 1 hour. Add celery and simmer 10 minutes. Add mushrooms, tofu, chicken and sesame oil and simmer 5–10 more minutes. Pour into bowls and garnish with green onion.

Calories per serving: 86
Calcium per serving: 73 mg

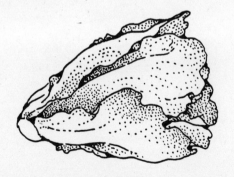

WATERCRESS SOUP

A light beginning to a Chinese dinner.

Number of servings: 5 ¾-cup servings

1 bunch watercress, washed and cut in thirds
2 14-ounce cans chicken broth
1 thin slice fresh ginger
2 green onions, thinly sliced

Combine watercress, broth and ginger in a 2-quart saucepan. Simmer for 15–20 minutes (or longer, if desired). Garnish each serving with green onion.

Calories per serving: 34
Calcium per serving: 46 mg

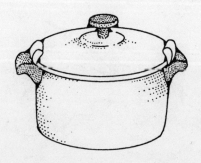

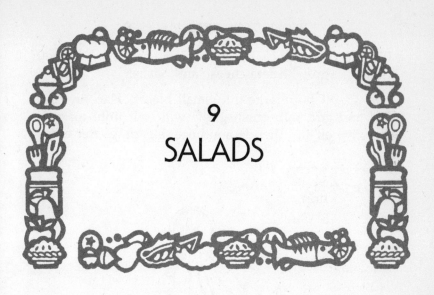

9
SALADS

GARLIC SALAD À LA RENA

Number of servings: 4

    4–5 cups romaine lettuce
    2 large tomatoes, sliced
    2 green onions, chopped
    ½ cup sliced fresh mushrooms
    4 ounces feta cheese, crumbled
    ¼ cup sliced black olives (optional)

Dressing:
    1 large or 2 small cloves garlic
    ¼–½ teaspoon salt
    1 teaspoon olive oil
    juice of ½ large lemon

Mix lettuce, tomatoes, onions and mushrooms. Toss with dressing. Top with feta cheese and olives.

Dressing: Chop garlic into small pieces. Place in small bowl and add salt; crush garlic with salt until mashed. Add olive oil and then lemon juice, blending after each.

Calories per serving: 130
Calcium per serving: 267 mg

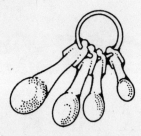

REFRESHING FRUIT SALAD

This unique fruit salad is sure to get rave reviews!

Number of servings: 6

> 1 8-ounce package Neufchâtel cheese, softened
> 1 cup cherry yogurt
> 1 tablespoon sugar
> ⅛ teaspoon vanilla
> ¼ teaspoon salt
> 1 16-ounce can pitted dark sweet cherries, drained
> 1 cup orange sections, cut in half
> 1 8-ounce can juice-packed crushed pineapple, drained
> ½ cup dried currants
> salad greens

Beat Neufchâtel cheese in large mixing bowl until smooth. Beat in yogurt, sugar, vanilla and salt on low speed. Set aside 6–12 cherries for garnish. Stir remaining cherries, orange, pineapple and currants into cheese mixture. Pour into a 4½-cup mold or six individual molds. Freeze at least 8 hours. Remove mold(s) from freezer and let stand at room temperature until softened, about 45–60 minutes for large mold. Unmold on salad greens. Garnish with reserved cherries.

Calories per serving: 265
Calcium per serving: 115 mg

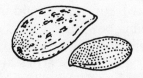

ALMOND-CARROT SALAD

Number of servings: 4 ¾-cup servings

3–4 medium carrots, finely shredded
½ cup chopped figs
¼ cup chopped almonds
¼ teaspoon salt
½ cup Cooked Salad Dressing, page 128

Mix all ingredients together in a bowl. Cover and refrigerate.

Calories per serving: 152
Calcium per serving: 102 mg

BLACKBERRY-ALMOND MOLD

Number of servings: 5

**1 cup canned blackberries, drained (reserve
    juice)**
**1 3-ounce package blackberry- or cherry-
    flavored gelatin**
1 cup vanilla yogurt
**⅓ cup slivered blanched almonds
    salad greens**

Add water to reserved liquid from canned berries, if necessary, to measure 1 cup. Boil liquid and combine with
gelatin in small mixing bowl until gelatin is dissolved. Cool.
Add yogurt and beat until smooth. Refrigerate until slightly
thickened but not set. Stir in berries and almonds. Pour
into 4-cup ring mold or 5 individual molds. Refrigerate
until firm. Unmold on salad greens.

Calories per serving: 202
Calcium per serving: 98 mg

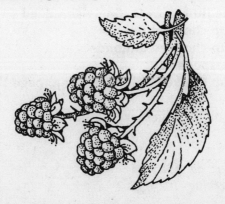

CAESAR SALAD

Serve with Shrimp and Cheese Soufflé and sourdough bread.

Number of servings: 6

>   1 egg
>   1 tablespoon olive oil
>   ¼ teaspoon garlic powder
>   1 cup cubed white bread, crust removed
>   1 medium clove garlic, crushed
>   ¼ teaspoon dry mustard
>   ½ teaspoon salt
>   ¼ teaspoon ground pepper
>   2 tablespoons olive oil
>   2 tablespoons water
> 1½ teaspoons Worcestershire sauce
>   8 anchovy fillets, drained and chopped
>   1 large bunch romaine lettuce, torn
>   ¼ cup grated Parmesan cheese
>   ¼ cup crumbled blue cheese
>   2 tablespoons lemon juice

Warm cold egg by immersing in warm water. In a small saucepan, boil enough water to cover egg completely. Immerse egg in boiling water with spoon; remove from heat. Cover and let stand 30 seconds. Immediately cool egg in cold water to prevent further cooking. Heat 1 tablespoon olive oil and garlic powder in nonstick skillet. Add bread cubes and sauté until browned, stirring often. Combine crushed garlic, mustard, salt, pepper, oil, water, Worcestershire sauce and anchovies in jar; cover and shake vigorously. Pour this dressing over lettuce in salad bowl, add cheeses and toss salad until it is well coated. Break egg into center of the salad. Pour lemon juice on top of egg and toss well. Add bread cubes, toss gently and serve immediately.

Calories per serving: 136
Calcium per serving: 143 mg

DOUBLE BEAN SALAD

If you don't like traditional bean salads, try this one! The combination of spices makes it one of a kind.

Number of servings: 8 ½-cup servings

> 1½ cups cooked or canned chickpeas (garbanzo beans), drained
> 1½ cups cooked or canned kidney beans, drained
> ¾ cup diced celery
> 1 tablespoon minced fresh cilantro
> 2 tablespoons minced fresh parsley
> ¾ cup Spicy Yogurt Dressing, page 131

Combine all ingredients in a salad bowl. Refrigerate before serving.

Calories per serving: 118
Calcium per serving: 97 mg

SALMON MACARONI SALAD

*This salad is a complete meal and can be served as a
main entrée or side dish.*

Number of servings: 18 ³/₄-cup servings

1 12-ounce package salad macaroni (about 2⅔
  cups dry
1 15½-ounce can salmon
1½ cups cooked whole-kernel corn
1½ cups finely chopped bell pepper (red and/or
  green)
½ cup chopped onion
¾ cup chopped jicama
  salt and pepper to taste
⅔ cup diet mayonnaise
⅔ cup plain yogurt
  paprika

Cook macaroni according to package directions, omitting
salt. Drain and cool. Drain salmon and break into chunks
in large bowl. Add macaroni, corn, bell pepper, onion,
jicama, salt and pepper, mixing well. Blend together mayonnaise and yogurt. Fold into salad ingredients. Place on
salad plates lined with spinach leaves. Sprinkle with paprika.

Calories per serving: 152
Calcium per serving: 74 mg

SALMON TOFU SALAD

A family favorite.

Number of servings: 6

> **1 14-ounce package firm tofu**
> **2 medium or large tomatoes, cubed**
> **1 7-ounce can salmon**
> **3 green onions, chopped**
> **1 tablespoon sesame seeds**

> *Sesame Dressing:*
> **4 tablespoons soy sauce**
> **2 tablespoons rice vinegar**
> **2 teaspoons sesame oil**
> **2 tablespoons white wine**

Drain water from tofu and cut tofu into cubes. Place in salad bowl. Arrange tomatoes over tofu, then shred salmon over mixture. Sprinkle with green onions and sesame seeds. Before serving, pour on Sesame Dressing.

Sesame Dressing: Pour ingredients into watertight container; shake well.

Calories per serving: 135
Calcium per serving: 168 mg

SPINACH SALAD

Number of servings: 8

> 2 tablespoons sesame seeds
> 1 pound fresh spinach
> 3 ounces (¾ cup) shredded cheddar cheese
> 2 green onions, sliced
> 1 15-ounce can unsweetened pineapple chunks, drained (reserve juice)
> 3 hard-cooked eggs, sliced
> 1 cup sliced mushrooms

Dressing:

> 1 tablespoon oil
> 4 tablespoons pineapple juice (reserved from canned chunks)
> 2 tablespoons white wine vinegar
> ½ teaspoon garlic salt
> ½ teaspoon ground ginger

Brown sesame seeds in nonstick skillet; set aside. Combine dressing ingredients in a jar. Cover and shake well to blend; refrigerate for several hours. Remove root ends and imperfect leaves from spinach. Wash spinach thoroughly; drain well, dry and tear leaves. Toss spinach, cheese, green onions and pineapple in a salad bowl. Garnish with eggs and mushrooms. Just before serving, shake dressing well, pour over salad and toss lightly. Sprinkle sesame seeds on top.

Calories per serving: 143
Calcium per serving: 143 mg

ZESTY BROCCOLI SALAD

Number of servings: 4 1-cup servings

> **2 10-ounce packages frozen broccoli flowerets**
> **2 ounces (½ cup) shredded sharp cheddar cheese**
> **4 tablespoons imitation bacon bits**
> **3 tablespoons diet mayonnaise**

Thaw broccoli thoroughly. Drain excess liquid, chop broccoli and transfer it to a salad bowl. Combine with cheese and bacon bits. Toss with mayonnaise. Cover and chill before serving.

Calories per serving: 140
Calcium per serving: 179 mg

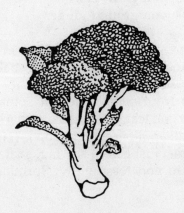

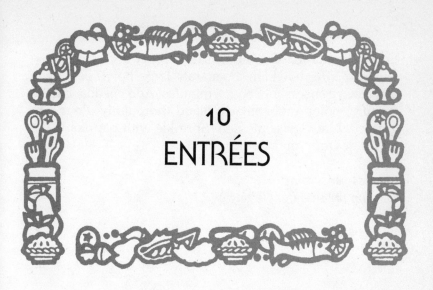

10
ENTRÉES

ANN'S SPECIAL SPINACH PIE

This crustless pie is very easy to make—and great for left-overs.

Number of servings: 6

> 8 ounces (2 cups) shredded sharp cheddar
>   cheese
> 5 tablespoons whole-wheat flour
> ¼ teaspoon salt
> ½ teaspoon pepper
> 1 teaspoon garlic powder
> 4 eggs
> 2 cups low-fat cottage cheese
> ½ cup chopped onion
> 1 10-ounce package frozen chopped spinach,
>   thawed and drained
>   paprika

Blend cheddar cheese, flour, salt, pepper and garlic powder in mixing bowl. In a separate large bowl, beat eggs
and cottage cheese for about 2 minutes. Add cheddar cheese
mixture, onion and spinach; blend thoroughly. Pour into
greased 9-inch glass pie pan. Sprinkle with paprika. Bake
at 350 degrees for 1 hour.

Calories per serving: 310
Calcium per serving: 407 mg

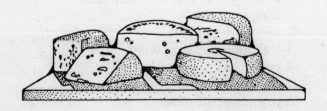

BAKED SOYBEANS

If you've never cooked with soybeans before, this is a great starter recipe: easy and delicious! Serve with a hearty bread and a salad for a complete meal.

Number of servings: 4 1-cup servings

> **10 ounces (about 1½ cups) dry soybeans, washed and picked over**
> **3¾ cups water (for soaking)**
> **water to cover beans**
> **1 8-ounce can tomato sauce**
> **1 large onion, chopped**
> **2 tablespoons molasses**
> **2 teaspoons oil**
> **3 tablespoons packed brown sugar**
> **¼ teaspoon dry mustard**
> **⅛ teaspoon pepper**
> **2 tablespoons imitation bacon bits**

Soak beans overnight in 3¾ cups water. Or, for short soak method, boil in 3¾ cups water for 2 minutes, then skim off loose bean-skins and let beans stand, covered, for 1 hour. Pour out water and add fresh water to cover. Heat to boiling; reduce heat. Cover and simmer until beans are soft and tender, not crunchy, at least 2 hours. Drain beans and place in a mixing bowl. Mix in other ingredients and pour into 1½-quart casserole. Cover and bake at 350 degrees 3–5 hours, stirring occasionally. Add extra water if beans become too dry.

Calories per serving: 360
Calcium per serving: 216 mg

BROCCOLI-STUFFED PASTA

Number of servings: 6

> 6 ounces (18–20) jumbo pasta shells
> 1 16-ounce bag frozen chopped broccoli, thawed
> 1 pound low-fat cottage cheese
> 8 ounces (2 cups) shredded part-skim mozzarella cheese
> ½ cup grated Parmesan cheese
> 1 tablespoon grated onion
> ½ teaspoon pepper
> 2 cloves crushed garlic or 1 teaspoon garlic powder
> 2 15½-ounce jars marinara sauce (or spaghetti sauce)

Cook pasta according to package directions. Drain. Combine broccoli, cottage cheese, 1½ cups mozzarella cheese, Parmesan cheese, onion, pepper and garlic. Fill shells with cheese-broccoli mixture. Spoon enough marinara sauce into bottom of 9 × 13-inch baking pan to cover bottom. Arrange shells in single layer; spoon remaining sauce over shells. Sprinkle rest of mozzarella cheese on top. Bake at 375 degrees until heated thoroughly, about 30 minutes. Cover the pan with foil for the first 15 minutes.

Calories per serving: 437
Calcium per serving: 493 mg

CHARLENE'S SPICY PORK TOFU

Number of servings: 4

> ¼ **pound zucchini**
> 1 **14-ounce block firm tofu**
> ¼ **pound ground pork**
> 1 **teaspoon minced garlic**
> 1 **teaspoon minced ginger**
> 1 **14-ounce can chicken broth**
> 2 **tablespoons cornstarch**
> 2 **tablespoons soy sauce**
> 1½ **tablespoons sugar**
> ½ **tablespoon chili sauce**
> 2 **tablespoons chopped green onion**

Cut zucchini and tofu into ½-inch-square cubes. Brown pork in a nonstick skillet. Add garlic, ginger and zucchini, cover and simmer until vegetable is tender. Combine remaining ingredients except onion and tofu in a small bowl. When vegetable is tender, uncover pan, increase heat to medium high and add chicken-broth mixture, stirring until sauce thickens. Boil and stir 1 minute. Gently fold in tofu and green onion. Heat thoroughly and serve.

Calories per serving: 205
Calcium per serving: 140 mg

CHEESY EGGPLANT PARMESAN

Number of servings: 6

> 1 large eggplant
> 1 28-ounce can tomato puree
> 2 teaspoons crumbled dry basil
> 1 teaspoon crumbled dry thyme
> 3 tablespoons finely chopped parsley
> 1½ teaspoons garlic powder
> ¼ teaspoon salt
> ⅛ teaspoon pepper
> 1 cup low-fat cottage cheese, drained
> 4 ounces (1 cup) shredded mozzarella cheese
> 4 ounces (1 cup) shredded Monterey Jack cheese
> ¼ cup grated Parmesan cheese, divided
> 1 tablespoon flour

Slice eggplant crosswide into ½-inch wheels. Steam for 10 minutes. Meanwhile, heat tomato puree, basil and thyme, and simmer to cook down. Mix together parsley, garlic powder, salt, pepper, cottage cheese, mozzarella and Monterey Jack cheeses, half of the Parmesan, and flour. In a 2-quart casserole, put layer of eggplant, then cheese mixture, then tomato sauce. Repeat layers. Top with remaining Parmesan cheese. Bake uncovered at 350 degrees for 30 minutes.

Calories per serving: 263
Calcium per serving: 383 mg

CHICKEN À LA QUEEN

This calcium-packed version of a traditional dish is fit for a queen.

Number of servings: 6 1½-cup servings

> **1 4-ounce can mushroom stems and pieces, drained (reserve liquid)**
> **1 small green pepper, chopped (about ½ cup)**
> **3 tablespoons margarine**
> **3 tablespoons cornstarch**
> **½ teaspoon salt**
> **¼ teaspoon pepper**
> **½ teaspoon ground marjoram**
> **1 chicken bouillon cube**
> **2¾ cups nonfat milk**
> **2 cups chicken, skinless, cooked and cut-up**
> **1 4-ounce jar whole pimientos, chopped**
> **4 cups Creamy Mashed Potatoes, page 110**

In a medium saucepan, cook and stir mushrooms and green pepper in margarine over medium heat for 5 minutes. Remove from heat. Sprinkle in cornstarch, salt, pepper and marjoram. Cook over low heat, stirring constantly, just until smooth; remove from heat. Stir in bouillon cube, milk and reserved mushroom liquid until smooth. Heat to boiling, stirring constantly. Boil and stir 1 minute. Stir in chicken and pimientos; heat thoroughly. Serve over mashed potatoes.

Calories per serving: 354
Calcium per serving: 255 mg

CHICKEN ENCHILADAS

Even the strictest waist-watcher will enjoy this low-fat version of a favorite Mexican dish.

Number of servings: 6

1½ chicken breasts, skinned
1¾ cups (14 fluid ounces) low-fat chicken broth (reserved)
¼ cup cornstarch
1 28-ounce can enchilada sauce
1 teaspoon sugar
1 teaspoon chili powder
12 corn tortillas
2 cups plain yogurt
2 ounces (½ cup) shredded part-skim mozzarella cheese
2 ounces (½ cup) diced low-calorie processed cheddar cheese
1 large onion, finely chopped
3 ounces (¾ cup) shredded cheddar cheese
3 ounces (¾ cup) shredded Monterey Jack cheese
2 green onions, chopped

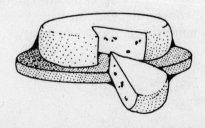

Cook chicken in water to cover until tender. Cool, then shred meat finely and discard bones. Reserve 1 ¾ cups broth. Dissolve cornstarch thoroughly in ½ cup enchilada sauce. Pour remaining enchilada sauce into a saucepan; blend in cornstarch mixture, sugar and chili powder. Soften tortillas by wrapping them in stacks of six in moistened (paper) towels and then in foil. Seal foil tightly; heat in 250-degree oven for 15 minutes. Beat yogurt with a fork until smooth; add small amount of broth to it until runny. Add yogurt and remaining reserved broth to enchilada-sauce mixture. Heat and stir over low-medium flame, adding in mozzarella and low-calorie cheddar cheeses and heating until melted. Do not boil. To assemble enchiladas, unwrap warmed tortillas. Place on each some of the chicken, onion, cheddar cheese and 1 tablespoon sauce. Roll and place seam side down in 9 × 13-inch baking pan. Top with sauce, using at least 2 cups. Sprinkle with Monterey Jack and remaining cheddar. Bake at 350 degrees until cheese is melted and sauce is bubbly, about 25–30 minutes. Top with green onions.

Calories per serving: 447
Calcium per serving: 617 mg

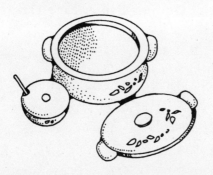

FALAFEL SANDWICHES WITH TAHINI SAUCE

A Middle Eastern delight.

Number of servings: 8 sandwiches

1 cup dried chickpeas (garbanzo beans)
5 cups water (for soaking)
  water to cover chickpeas
2 cloves garlic, finely minced
½ teaspoon salt
½ cup very finely minced onion
2 tablespoons very finely minced parsley
1 tablespoon very finely minced cilantro
1 teaspoon ground cumin
1 tablespoon lemon juice
  dash black pepper
⅛ teaspoon cayenne pepper
1 teaspoon olive oil
1 teaspoon baking soda
8 pita-bread pockets
4 tomatoes, sliced
8 ounces (2 cups) shredded cheddar cheese
2 cups shredded lettuce
  Tahini Dipping Sauce, page 133

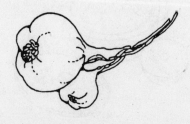

Soak chickpeas in 5 cups water overnight. Drain water, rinse beans and replace with water to cover. Simmer beans about 35–45 minutes or until tender. Meanwhile, crush garlic with salt, then mix with onion, parsley, cilantro, cumin, lemon juice, black pepper, cayenne pepper and oil. Drain chickpeas and put them with the baking soda into a blender or food processor. Blend until chickpeas are the texture of coarse bread crumbs (not a paste). Combine chickpeas with the seasoning mixture. Form into 20–22 patties 1¾ inches in diameter, ¾ inch thick in the middle and less thick at the edges. Place on cookie sheet and bake in 350-degree oven for about 15 minutes. To assemble sandwiches, put 2 or 3 patties into each pita-bread pocket. Add tomato slices, shredded cheese and lettuce, and top with 2 tablespoons Tahini Dipping Sauce.

Calories per serving: 349
Calcium per serving: 283 mg

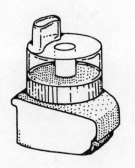

GARDEN BURRITO

Number of servings: 1

> **1 8-inch flour tortilla**
> **½ cup canned, drained pinto beans**
> **1 cup shredded lettuce**
> **1 tomato, chopped**
> **1 tablespoon chopped onion**
> **2 ounces (½ cup) shredded cheddar or**
> **Monterey Jack cheese**
> **salsa to taste**

Warm flour tortilla in oven or microwave. Mash beans with potato masher or fork and heat over medium flame, stirring occasionally. Spread beans on tortilla. Top with lettuce, tomato, onion, cheese and salsa.

Calories per serving: 527
Calcium per serving: 551 mg

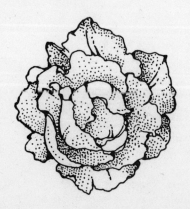

ITALIAN PASTA SALAD

A meal in itself.

Number of servings: 14 1½-cup servings

> 1 1-pound box small shells
> ¼ pound each of ham, salami and pepperoni, cut up
> ½ pound each of mozzarella and Muenster cheeses, cut up
> 3 green peppers, diced
> 4 tomatoes, diced
> 3 green onions, chopped
> 4 stalks celery, diced
> ½ cup sliced black olives

Dressing:
> ½ cup vegetable or salad oil
> ½ cup white vinegar
> ¼ cup white wine
> ½ teaspoon oregano
> 2 cloves garlic, crushed

Cook shells according to package instructions. Rinse with cold water, drain and cool. Mix pasta with other ingredients and toss with dressing.

Dressing: Place all ingredients in a watertight jar. Shake well.

Calories per serving: 398
Calcium per serving: 259 mg

MEXICAN QUICHE

The crust used in this quiche is lower in fat and calories than regular pie crust.

Number of servings: 6

> 1 cup buttermilk baking mix
> 4 tablespoons plus 1 teaspoon cold water
> 1 cup evaporated nonfat milk
> 3 eggs, slightly beaten
> ⅛ teaspoon ground cumin
> 3 ounces (¾ cup) shredded part-skim mozzarella cheese
> 2 ounces (½ cup) shredded Monterey Jack cheese
> 5 ounces (1¼ cup) shredded cheddar cheese, divided
> 1 4-ounce can diced green chilies, drained

Preheat oven to 425 degrees. Mix together baking mix and water until dough forms. With floured hands pat dough into deep-dish 9-inch pie pan and bake for about 10 minutes or until pale gold. Beat milk, eggs and cumin until blended. Sprinkle mozzarella and Monterey Jack and half the cheddar over bottom of pan. Distribute chilies over cheese, then pour milk mixture into shell. Sprinkle with remaining cheddar. Bake at 325 degrees 55–60 minutes or until center of pie is set (shake gently to test). Let stand for 15 minutes before cutting.

Calories per serving: 329
Calcium per serving: 476 mg

MICHIGAN MEATLOAF

Number of servings: 10 3³/₄-ounce servings

2 pounds ground round beef
2 eggs
1 cup nonfat dry milk
1 medium onion, diced
½ cup Italian-style bread crumbs
2 teaspoons salt
½ teaspoon garlic powder

Blend all ingredients well; form into a loaf. Bake in loaf pan or roasting pan, covered, at 350 degrees for about 1½ hours.

Calories per serving: 212
Calcium per serving: 106 mg

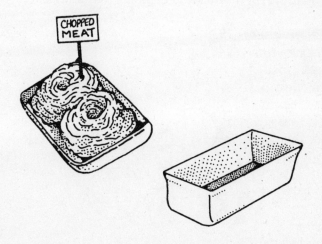

ORIENTAL OMELET

Number of servings: 3

> 9–10 ounces firm tofu, drained and finely cubed
> 3 eggs, lightly beaten
> 1 tablespoon soy sauce
> ¼ teaspoon honey
> 1 tablespoon sesame oil
> 3 large fresh mushrooms, sliced
> 2 green onions, chopped

Combine first four ingredients in a large bowl and mix well. Heat oil in a large nonstick skillet. Add mushrooms and green onion, and sauté 2–3 minutes, until slightly cooked. Add mushrooms and onions to tofu-egg mixture and stir. Pour mixture back into skillet and cook over low heat, lifting gently at sides to allow uncooked egg to flow underneath. When omelet is cooked, fold and serve.

Calories per serving: 193
Calcium per serving: 149 mg

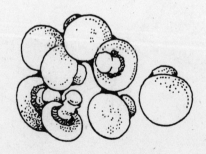

OYSTERS PARMESAN

Number of servings: 4

> 1 tablespoon olive oil
> 1 large onion, chopped
> ½ teaspoon thyme leaves
> ¼ teaspoon ground oregano
> 3 cloves garlic, finely chopped
> 3 tablespoons chopped parsley
> ¼ teaspoon red pepper sauce
>   salt to taste
>   pepper to taste
> 1 pound (1 pint) chucked oysters with liquor
> 1 cup Italian-style bread crumbs
> ⅔ cup grated Parmesan cheese

Heat oil in a nonstick skillet. Add onion and sauté until limp. Add all of the seasonings and mix well. Add oysters; heat over medium flame for several minutes. Add liquor. Fold in the bread crumbs. Transfer the mixture to a greased casserole. Sprinkle the dish with Parmesan cheese. Bake at 350 degrees for about 20 minutes.

Calories per serving: 281
Calcium per serving: 337 mg

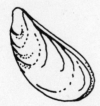
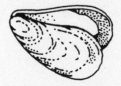

PINEAPPLE CHICKEN

Number of servings: 6

> 2 ounces sliced unsalted almonds
> 1 large onion, diced
> 2 12-ounce cans nonfat evaporated milk
> 1 4-ounce can sliced mushrooms
> 1 teaspoon salt
> ½ teaspoon pepper
> ⅛ teaspoon powdered ginger
> 1 16-ounce can unsweetened pineapple
>   chunks, drained
> 2 teaspoons cornstarch
> 2⅓ cups cooked skinless chicken, cubed
> 4 cups cooked rice
>   parsley

Brown almonds in nonstick skillet. Remove almonds, and brown onion until tender. (Add a little water to pan, if needed.) To onion add all but ½ cup of the milk, mushrooms, salt, pepper, ginger and pineapple. Stir over medium heat until hot. Add cornstarch to reserved milk and blend. Add chicken, almonds and cornstarch mixture to sauce and bring to a boil, stirring constantly. Boil 1 minute. Serve over rice. Garnish with parsley.

Calories per serving: 457
Calcium per serving: 427 mg

POACHED SOLE WITH SHRIMP SAUCE

Serve with steamed rice.

Number of servings: 4

> 1 tablespoon margarine
> 6 ounces (about 2½ cups) fresh, sliced mushrooms
> juice of ½ lemon
> salt
> white pepper
> 1 pound (about 6 fillets) Dover sole
> ½ cup dry white wine
> 1 bay leaf
> ¼ pound small cooked shrimp
> 1 cup White Wine Sauce, page 136
> parsley

Melt margarine in skillet and add mushrooms, lemon juice and dash salt. Heat and stir until mushrooms are browned. Remove mushrooms and set aside. Use salt and pepper to season fish, and fold each fillet in half. Arrange in one layer in skillet. Add wine and bay leaf, cover and poach gently until fish flakes easily, about 8–10 minutes. Meanwhile, stir mushrooms and shrimp into White Wine Sauce, and heat thoroughly over low flame. When fish is cooked, carefully lift it from skillet to hot platter. Pour sauce over poached fish and garnish with parsley.

Calories per serving: 229
Calcium per serving: 237 mg

RECIPES FOR BETTER BONES

SALMON-TOFU PATTIES

As easy and delicious as hamburgers, these patties provide the perfect introduction for the tofuphobic cook.

Number of servings: 6 patties

**1 14-ounce block firm tofu
1 7-ounce can salmon, drained and cut up
2 egg whites
3 green onions, finely chopped
⅛ teaspoon black pepper**

Squeeze water from tofu in cheesecloth. Break up tofu into small pieces and blend with salmon, using a fork or food processor. Add other ingredients and mix well. Form hamburger-size patties. Brown in nonstick pan, about 5 minutes on each side.

Calories per serving: 124
Calcium per serving: 139 mg

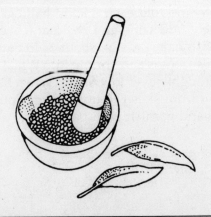

SHRIMP AND CHEESE SOUFFLÉ

Number of servings: 4

- ⅓ **cup nonfat dry milk**
- 1 **cup nonfat milk**
- 2 **tablespoons margarine**
- 2 **tablespoons cornstarch**
- 3 **ounces low-calorie processed cheddar cheese**
- 3 **eggs, separated**
- ¼ **teaspoon cream of tartar**
- 1 **4½-ounce can tiny shrimp, rinsed and drained**
- ½ **teaspoon dried basil leaves**
- 1 **teaspoon dried tarragon leaves**

Blend dry milk into liquid milk until smooth; set aside. Heat oven to 350 degrees. Grease soufflé dish or 1½-quart casserole. Melt margarine in saucepan over low heat. Blend in cornstarch, stirring constantly, until mixture is smooth and bubbly; remove from heat. Stir in milk. Heat to boiling, stirring constantly. Stir in cheese until melted; remove from heat. Beat egg whites and cream of tartar until stiff but not dry. Beat egg yolks until very thick, about 5 minutes. Add shrimp, basil, tarragon and egg yolks to cheese mixture, stirring after each. Stir one-fourth of the egg whites into cheese mixture. Fold cheese mixture into remaining egg whites. Pour carefully into soufflé dish. Cook uncovered until knife inserted halfway between center and edge comes out clean, 50–60 minutes.

Calories per serving: 236
Calcium per serving: 359 mg

TASTY STUFFED TROUT

Number of servings: 4

> ⅔ cup minced celery
> 1 ounce (about 8 fillets) canned anchovies, minced (reserve 2 teaspoons oil)
> 1 egg
> ¾ cup Italian-style bread crumbs
> 4 tablespoons Parmesan cheese
> ½ cup nonfat dry milk
> ¼ cup chopped parsley
> 2 tablespoons lemon juice
> 4 drawn whole trout (6–8 ounces each)
> salt
> pepper
> cherry tomatoes (optional)
> parsley (optional)

Cook celery in nonstick pan with anchovies and oil until tender. Empty into mixing bowl. Stir in egg, bread crumbs, cheese, dry milk, parsley and lemon juice. Rub cavities of trout with salt and pepper; stuff each with bread-crumb mixture. Place fish in greased 9 × 13-inch baking dish. Bake uncovered at 350 degrees until fish flakes easily with fork, 30–35 minutes. Garnish with cherry tomatoes and snipped parsley, if desired.

Calories per serving: 515
Calcium per serving: 605 mg

TOFU VEGETABLES

Number of servings: 6 1-cup servings

¼ cup low-sodium soy sauce
1 tablespoon sugar
½ teaspoon garlic powder
1 tablespoon cornstarch
1 14-ounce block firm tofu, drained and cut into ¾-inch cubes
½ cup chicken or beef broth
2 stalks (about ⅔ cup) sliced celery
3 green onions, sliced
½ cup chopped green pepper
¼ pound (about 1½ cups) sliced mushrooms
½ cup sliced water chestnuts
½ cup bamboo shoots
¼ pound snow peas
½ cup sliced almonds
¼ pound bean sprouts

Mix soy sauce, sugar and garlic powder together in a flat-bottomed container until dissolved. Blend in cornstarch until smooth. Add tofu and marinate for several hours, turning occasionally. In a large nonstick skillet or wok bring broth to a boil. Add celery, onions and pepper and simmer for 3 minutes, stirring occasionally. Add mushrooms, water chestnuts, bamboo shoots and snow peas, and simmer for 2 minutes. Stir in tofu cubes and almonds; simmer for 2 minutes. Add bean sprouts and pour remainder of soy sauce mixture over all. Stir for 1 minute. Serve immediately.

Calories per serving: 167
Calcium per serving: 121 mg

TURKEY TACO CASSEROLE

Number of servings: 12

8 6-inch corn tortillas
1¾ pounds ground turkey
1 onion, chopped
2 cloves garlic, pressed
1½ teaspoons chili powder
¼ teaspoon ground cumin
¼ teaspoon thyme
¼ teaspoon salt
½ teaspoon oregano
1 pound Monterey Jack cheese, shredded
6 eggs
2 cups nonfat milk
1 cup plain yogurt
3 tomatoes, chopped
3 cups shredded lettuce
olives (optional)
salsa (optional)

Line greased 9 × 13-inch baking dish with tortillas, tearing to fit and putting in two layers. In large skillet, brown turkey and onion, draining off fat. Add garlic, chili powder, cumin, thyme, salt and oregano. Pour into baking dish. Top with cheese. In bowl, beat eggs with milk and pour over ingredients in baking dish. Bake at 350 degrees for 1 hour, until custard sets. While still warm, spread with yogurt, then tomatoes, lettuce and olives, if desired. Pass salsa at table, if desired.

Calories per serving: 378
Calcium per serving: 437 mg

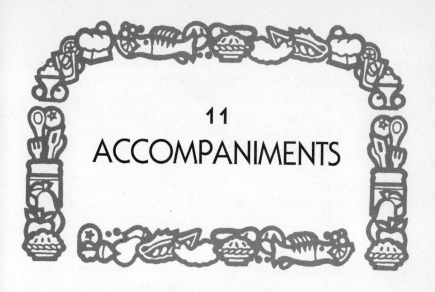

11
ACCOMPANIMENTS

CHEESY NOODLE SCALLOP

Number of servings: 8

4 cups wide noodles, cooked
2 tablespoons cornstarch
2 cups nonfat milk
½ cup finely chopped onion
½ cup finely chopped green pepper
1 tablespoon margarine
½ teaspoon celery seed
8 ounces feta cheese, crumbled
⅔ cup low-fat cottage cheese
paprika

Cook noodles according to package instructions. Drain well and set aside. Add cornstarch to ½ cup milk in a small container and mix well. Set aside. In a saucepan cook onion and green pepper in margarine until tender. Stir in celery seed. Slowly add remainder of milk and the cornstarch mixture and cook over medium flame until thickened, stirring constantly until boiling. Boil and stir 1 minute. Fold in feta and cottage cheese. Combine noodles and sauce and turn into a greased 2-quart casserole. Sprinkle with paprika. Bake uncovered at 350 degrees for 45 minutes.

Calories per serving: 247
Calcium per serving: 320 mg

CREAMY MASHED POTATOES

Number of servings: 8 ³/₄-cup servings

> **2 pounds (about 6 medium) potatoes**
> **about ½ cup nonfat milk**
> **½ cup nonfat dry milk**
> **2 ounces (¼ cup) cream cheese, softened**
> **½ teaspoon salt**
> **dash pepper**
> **½ teaspoon dill weed (optional)**
> **parsley or chives (optional)**

Wash and pare potatoes; remove any eyes. Cut potatoes into large pieces. Heat 1 inch of water to boiling in saucepan. Add potatoes, cover and heat to boiling. Cook until tender, 20–25 minutes; drain thoroughly. Shake pan gently over low heat to dry potatoes. Mash potatoes until no lumps remain. Beat in liquid milk and dry milk in small amounts, alternating the two. (Amount of liquid milk needed depends on type of potatoes used and consistency desired.) Add cream cheese, salt, pepper and dill, if desired.

Beat until potatoes are light and fluffy. Sprinkle with snipped parsley or chives, if desired.

Calories per serving: 156
Calcium per serving: 91 mg

GNOCCHI

Number of servings: 8

> **3 cups nonfat milk**
> **1 cup uncooked farina (Cream of Wheat)**
> **2 eggs, well beaten**
> **2 tablespoons cream cheese**
> **1 teaspoon garlic salt**
>   **dash pepper**
> **1 tablespoon margarine**
> **⅔ cup grated Parmesan cheese**

Heat milk to scalding in 2-quart saucepan; reduce heat. Sprinkle farina slowly into hot milk, stirring constantly. Cook until thick, about 5 minutes, stirring constantly. (Spoon will stand upright when mixture is ready.) Remove from heat. Stir in eggs, cream cheese, garlic salt and pepper; beat until smooth. Spread into greased 13 × 9-inch pan; cool. Cover and refrigerate until firm, 2–3 hours. Cut dough into 1½-inch circles. (Dip knife in cold water to prevent sticking.) Place circles, overlapping, in ungreased baking dish. Dot with margarine; sprinkle with Parmesan cheese. Bake uncovered in 350-degree oven until crisp and golden, about 45 minutes.

Calories per serving: 186
Calcium per serving: 337 mg

ITALIAN RICE AND PEAS

Number of servings: 8

- ½ cup chopped onion
- 1⅓ cups dry brown rice
- 2⅔ cups water
- 2 chicken bouillon cubes
- 1 10-ounce package frozen peas, cooked and drained
- ¾ cup grated Parmesan cheese

Brown onion and rice in a nonstick skillet, stirring occasionally. Stir in water and bouillon cubes, and bring to a boil, stirring once or twice. Set the heat as low as possible, cover and simmer until the rice is tender and the liquid is absorbed, about 30–40 minutes. Remove from heat. Gently fold in peas; cover and let set for 5–10 minutes. Stir in cheese lightly; serve.

Calories per serving: 188
Calcium per serving: 125 mg

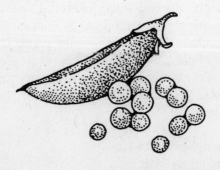

OYSTER STUFFING

This light side dish won't leave you "stuffed"—it has no added fat!

Number of servings: 4 1-cup servings

> ¾ cup finely chopped onion
> ¾ cup chopped celery, with leaves
> 4 cups soft bread cubes
> ⅔ cup nonfat evaporated milk
> 1 8-ounce can oysters, drained and chopped
> 1 teaspoon salt
> ¾ teaspoon dried sage leaves
> ½ teaspoon dried thyme leaves
> ¼ teaspoon pepper

Cook and stir onion and celery in nonstick pan until onion is tender. Mix all ingredients together in a large mixing bowl. Turn into greased 1½-quart casserole, cover and bake at 325 degrees for 1 hour. Uncover for the last 15 minutes to brown, if desired.

Calories per serving: 149
Calcium per serving: 203 mg

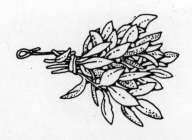

POTATO CASSEROLE

Number of servings: 8 1-cup servings

> **2 pounds (about 6 medium) potatoes**
> **pepper**
> **1 teaspoon garlic salt**
> **3 tablespoons chopped parsley**
> **1 small onion, chopped (about ¼ cup)**
> **4 ounces (about 1 cup) thinly sliced or**
> **shredded low-calorie processed cheddar**
> **cheese**
> **1 cup evaporated whole milk**

Wash and pare potatoes, removing any eyes. Cut into lengthwise strips, ¼–³⁄₈-inch wide. Arrange potatoes in greased 2-quart casserole in 3 layers, topping each layer with a dash of pepper and one-third each of the garlic salt, parsley, onion and cheese. Pour milk over potatoes. Cover and cook at 350 degrees until potatoes are tender, about 60–70 minutes.

Calories per serving: 200
Calcium per serving: 197 mg

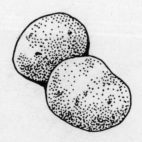

SPECIAL STUFFED POTATOES

A delicious complement to a classic entrée, such as poached fish or prime rib.

Number of servings: 6

> **4 green onions, chopped**
> **¼ pound (about 1½ cups) fresh sliced mushrooms**
> **⅔ cup evaporated nonfat milk**
> **4 ounces (1 cup) shredded Swiss cheese**
> **4 ounces (about ⅔ cup) crumbled feta cheese**
> **1 4½-ounce can small shrimp, drained**
> **6 baked potatoes with pulp spooned out and reserved**
> **¼ teaspoon salt**
> **⅛ teaspoon cayenne pepper**
> **paprika**

Steam green onions and mushrooms with small amount of water in nonstick pan until tender and mushrooms are browned. Remove from heat and add milk. Whisk in cheese a little at a time over low flame. When cheese is melted, stir in shrimp. Mix in pulp from potatoes, salt and cayenne pepper. Refill potato skins with mixture. Sprinkle with paprika. Broil 3 minutes.

Calories per serving: 318
Calcium per serving: 440 mg

SUNSET SURPRISE

Number of servings: 12 3 × 3¼-inch pieces

> 27 single graham crackers
> 5 tablespoons (⅔ stick) margarine, softened
> 2⅔ tablespoons sugar
> 1 3-ounce box strawberry gelatin
> 1 cup hot water
> 1 pound low-fat cottage cheese
> 1 cup sugar
> ½ cup evaporated whole milk, chilled
> 2 teaspoons lemon juice
> 4 teaspoons sugar
> 1 teaspoon vanilla
> *Also needed:*
> > chilled mixing bowl
> > chilled beaters

Crush crackers with rolling pin or in blender or food processor. Mix crackers with margarine and 2⅔ tablespoons sugar until fine crumbs are formed. Pat into the bottom of a 13 × 9-inch cake pan but reserve a little for the top. Dissolve gelatin in hot water and let partly jell. Beat cottage cheese with 1 cup sugar. When gelatin is ready, pour milk into chilled bowl and beat with chilled beaters until foamy. Add lemon juice and beat until firm; add 4 teaspoons sugar and vanilla and beat until stiff. Mix gelatin with cottage cheese, then carefully fold in whipped milk. Pour into pan. Sprinkle with reserved crumbs. Refrigerate before serving.

Calories per serving: 261
Calcium per serving: 62 mg

TEX-MEX RICE AND CHEESE

Number of servings: 8 1-cup servings

> **3 cups cooked rice**
> **2 cups plain yogurt**
> **1½ teaspoons garlic salt**
> **1 teaspoon onion powder**
> **8 ounces (2 cups) shredded Monterey Jack cheese, divided**
> **1 6-ounce can whole peeled chilies, drained and chopped, divided**

Combine rice, yogurt, garlic salt and onion powder. Arrange half of rice mixture in a greased 2-quart casserole. Top with half of the cheese and chilies, then the rest of the rice mixture, and finally with the remainder of the cheese and chilies. Bake at 325 degrees for 30 minutes.

Calories per serving: 226
Calcium per serving: 319 mg

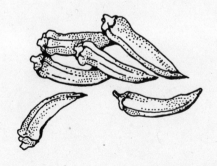

TWO-STEP RICE AND BEANS

A savory side dish to quesadillas or Spanish omelettes.

Number of servings: 6 1-cup servings

> 1 cup chopped onion
> 2 15-ounce cans pinto beans, drained
> 2 cups cooked rice
> 8 ounces tomato sauce
> 3 tablespoons imitation bacon bits
> ¼ cup packed brown sugar
> 1 teaspoon prepared mustard
> 1½ teaspoons salt
> ¼ teaspoon black pepper

Cook onion in nonstick skillet until tender but not browned. Stir in all other ingredients. Cover and simmer for about 10 minutes.

Calories per serving: 257
Calcium per serving: 66 mg

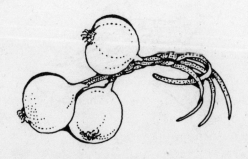

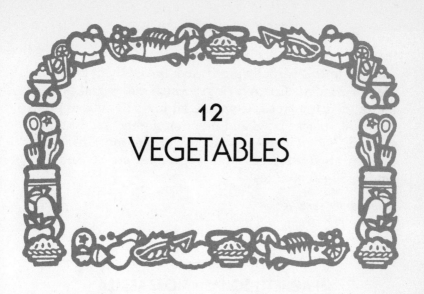

12
VEGETABLES

COLORFUL VEGETABLE BAKE

Number of servings: 12 ½-cup servings

> 1 cup sliced carrots, fresh or frozen, thawed
> and drained
> 1½ cups sliced green beans, fresh or frozen,
> thawed and drained
> 1 14-ounce block firm tofu, drained
> 1 1-pound can whole tomatoes, drained
> 1 cup corn, fresh or frozen, thawed and
> drained
> 2 cloves garlic, minced
> ½ teaspoon salt
> dash pepper
> ¼ cup slivered almonds

If fresh carrots and green beans are used, they will be crunchy unless partially precooked. Steam them for 5 minutes, if desired. Cut tofu into ½-inch cubes and quarter the canned tomatoes. Combine all ingredients except almonds in a large bowl and mix thoroughly. Transfer into greased 2-quart casserole. Top with almonds. Bake uncovered at 375 degrees until vegetables are cooked and tender, 30–40 minutes.

Calories per serving: 64
Calcium per serving: 69 mg

SPAGHETTI-SQUASH MOZZARELLA

Spaghetti squash is a large oblong yellow summer squash that separates into spaghetti-like strands after it's cooked.

Number of servings: 8 ½-cup servings

> ½ spaghetti squash, cut lengthwise
> 2 ounces (½ cup) shredded part-skim
>   mozzarella cheese
> 1 tablespoon grated Parmesan cheese
> 3 tablespoons seasoned dry bread crumbs
> 1 teaspoon garlic powder
> 1 tablespoon chopped parsley

Clean out seeds from squash. Place squash, cut side down, in a pot with 2 inches water; cover and boil for 20 minutes. Completely scoop out strands of cooked squash into a bowl by running fork over inside. In another bowl combine remaining ingredients and mix well. Add this mixture to bowl with squash and blend. Place in casserole dish and bake uncovered at 350 degrees until slightly browned and cheese melts, about 20 minutes.

Calories per serving: 42
Calcium per serving: 82 mg

BOK CHOY WITH MUSHROOMS

Also known as Chinese mustard cabbage, bok choy has large dark green leaves and long white stems. The stalks are stringless, crunchy and mild in flavor.

Number of servings: 6 ½-cup servings

> 1¼ **pounds bok choy**
> 1 **chicken bouillon cube**
> ¾ **cup boiling water**
> 1 **tablespoon cornstarch**
> 1 **teaspoon sugar**
> ¼ **teaspoon powdered ginger**
> 1 **tablespoon soy sauce**
> 1 **tablespoon margarine**
> ½ **cup chopped onion**
> ¼ **pound (about 1½ cups) sliced mushrooms**
> 1 **medium (¾ cup) carrot, sliced diagonally**
> 1 **clove garlic, minced**

Cut bok choy lengthwise through stalk and then crosswise in ¼- to ½-inch slices. Combine bouillon and water to make broth; mix cornstarch, sugar, ginger, soy sauce and half of the broth. Melt margarine in nonstick wok or large skillet and add onion. Sauté for 2 minutes. Add mushrooms and sauté for another 2 minutes. Remove from wok and set aside. Add bok choy, carrot, garlic and the unmixed broth to wok and stir-fry for 2 minutes. Stir in cornstarch-broth mixture. Cook and stir until mixture boils and thickens. Reduce heat and simmer, covered, until vegetables are tender, about 3 minutes. Return mushrooms to wok. Heat until hot.

Calories per serving: 58
Calcium per serving: 168 mg

BROCCOLI STIR-FRY

A classic Chinese dish.

Number of servings: 4 ½-cup servings

1 pound broccoli
1 tablespoon vegetable oil
1 garlic clove, crushed
½ teaspoon salt
1 teaspoon rice wine or dry sherry
¼ teaspoon sugar
3 tablespoons chicken broth
¼ cup water

Rinse broccoli with cold water. Cut into 2-inch flowerets and slice stems ¼ inch thick. Heat oil in a nonstick skillet or wok over high heat for 30 seconds. Stir-fry garlic until golden, about 30 seconds. Add broccoli stems and salt. Stir-fry for 30 seconds. Add broccoli flowerets. Stir-fry 1 minute. Add wine, sugar, broth and water. Reduce heat to medium-low and continue to stir-fry until water is almost gone. Serve hot.

Calories per serving: 53
Calcium per serving: 69 mg

CREAMED TURNIP GREENS

Number of servings: 12 ¹/₂-cup servings

> 1 large onion, chopped
> 2 stalks celery, chopped
> 1¹/₂ pounds fresh turnip greens
> 1 tablespoon cornstarch
> 1 12-ounce can evaporated nonfat milk
> 1 teaspoon garlic powder
> ¹/₂ teaspoon salt
> 1 teaspoon sugar
> dash pepper
> 2 tablespoons imitation bacon bits

Cook onion and celery in nonstick pan until tender; set aside. Remove root ends and imperfect leaves from turnip greens; wash thoroughly. Cook greens, covered, in small amount of water until tender, about 15–20 minutes. Meanwhile, blend cornstarch into milk; add garlic powder, salt, sugar and pepper. Cook over low flame, stirring constantly, until thickened (to the consistency of condensed canned cream soup). Drain greens and combine with milk mixture, onion and celery. Turn into ungreased 8-inch-square baking dish (or similar size). Sprinkle bacon bits on top. Cook uncovered in 350-degree oven until browned, about 25–30 minutes.

Calories per serving: 58
Calcium per serving: 196 mg

SALTED SPINACH SAUTÉ

Number of servings: 3

> **1 pound fresh spinach**
> **1 ounce canned anchovies, chopped**
> **1 small onion, thinly sliced**
> **dash pepper**

Remove root ends and imperfect leaves from spinach. Wash thoroughly and drain. Cook and stir anchovies with onion in large nonstick skillet until onion is tender. Add about half the spinach, and the pepper. Cover and cook over medium heat for 2 minutes, adding a little water if necessary. Add remaining spinach. Cover and cook, stirring occasionally, until spinach is tender, 3–10 minutes.

Calories per serving: 47
Calcium per serving: 108 mg

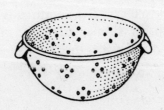

SPICY COLLARDS

This serves as an alternative to potato or garden salad.

Number of servings: 6 ½-cup servings

> **2 teaspoons olive oil**
> **1 medium onion, finely chopped**
> **2 cloves garlic, mashed**
> **¼ cup finely minced fresh parsley**
> **1 teaspoon sugar**
> **1 16-ounce package frozen chopped collard greens**
> **1½ cups plain yogurt**
> **1 teaspoon salt**
> **⅓ cup bulgur wheat**

Heat the oil in a medium nonstick pan. Add the onion and sauté over medium flame until soft. Add the garlic and stir for 15 seconds. Next add parsley and stir for another 15 seconds. Remove from heat and let cool. Add sugar to greens and cook according to package directions. Rinse cooked greens under cold water, squeeze out as much liquid as possible and mince. Place yogurt in a bowl and beat with a fork until smooth. Add onion mixture, collard greens, salt and bulgur; mix thoroughly.

Calories per serving: 93
Calcium per serving: 218 mg

SWISS VEGETABLES

This colorful and tasty combination might even appeal to the vegetable haters in your family.

Number of servings: 8 ½-cup servings

> 1 tablespoon cornstarch
> 10 ounces evaporated nonfat milk
> 1 16-ounce bag frozen broccoli-carrot-and-cauliflower combination, thawed and drained
> 1 4-ounce can mushrooms, drained
> 3 ounces (¾ cup) shredded Swiss cheese
> ½ cup seasoned bread crumbs, divided
> ⅓ cup plain yogurt
> ¼ teaspoon salt
> ¼ teaspoon pepper

Add cornstarch to milk slowly and blend thoroughly. Cook in saucepan over low heat until boiling, stirring constantly. Stir and boil 1 minute. Add vegetables and mushrooms to milk mixture; add ½ cup cheese, ¼ cup bread crumbs, yogurt, salt and pepper, and blend well. Pour into 1½-quart casserole. Bake covered at 350 degrees for 30 minutes. Mix remaining cheese and bread crumbs and sprinkle on top of casserole. Bake uncovered 5 minutes longer.

Calories per serving: 121
Calcium per serving: 262 mg

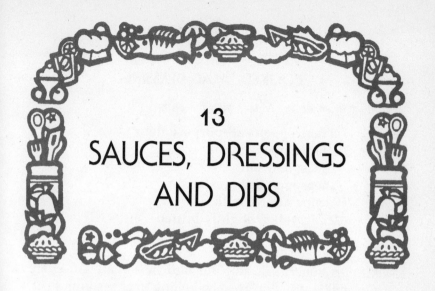

13
SAUCES, DRESSINGS AND DIPS

BLUE CHEESE DIP

Number of servings: Makes 4 cups

> 2½ cups plain yogurt
> 1½ cups low-calorie mayonnaise
> ½ cup chopped onion
> 6 ounces blue cheese, finely crumbled
>   pinch salt
> ½ teaspoon garlic powder
> 1–2 tablespoons chopped parsley

Mix yogurt and mayonnaise. Add other ingredients and mix well. Serve cold with cut raw vegetables or crackers or as a salad dressing. Dip can also be heated in a microwave and served with baked corn tortillas or tortilla chips.

Calories per serving: 24 per tablespoon
Calcium per serving: 32 mg per tablespoon

COOKED SALAD DRESSING

Number of servings: Makes about 2 cups

5 tablespoons all-purpose flour
1½ tablespoons sugar
1 teaspoon salt
1 teaspoon dry mustard
1½ cups nonfat milk
2 egg yolks, slightly beaten
⅓ cup rice vinegar

Mix flour, sugar, salt and mustard in 2-quart saucepan. Stir in milk gradually. Heat to boiling over medium heat, stirring constantly. Boil and stir 1 minute. Gradually stir at least half of the hot mixture into egg yolks, then blend back into the rest of the hot mixture in saucepan. Boil and stir 1 minute. Remove from heat; stir in vinegar. Cool slightly; refrigerate.

Calories per serving: 17 per tablespoon
Calcium per serving: 20 mg per tablespoon

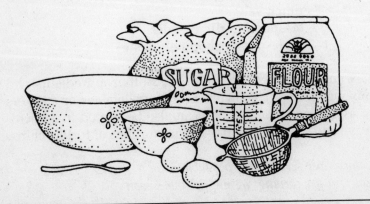

CLAM SAUCE

Number of servings: 4 side-dish servings

> 2 6½-ounce cans chopped clams
> ⅔ cup clam juice (reserved from canned clams)
> ½ tablespoon cornstarch
> 1 tablespoon olive oil
> 1 tablespoon margarine
> 1 small onion, minced
> 2 small cloves garlic, minced
>   salt to taste
>   white pepper to taste
> ¼ teaspoon oregano

Drain clams, reserving ⅔ cup juice; add cornstarch to juice and blend well. Put oil, margarine, onion, garlic, salt and pepper in pan and cook until golden. Add oregano, drained clams and clam juice. Stir over low heat until thickened. Turn up heat and bring sauce to a boil. Boil 1 minute. Serve hot over 2–2½ cups cooked linguine; sprinkle with chopped parsley and Parmesan cheese.

Calories per serving: 129
Calcium per serving: 75 mg

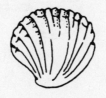

LIGHT ITALIAN DIP

Number of servings: makes 1½ cups

1 3-ounce package cream cheese, softened
1 cup plain yogurt
1 envelope low-calorie Italian dressing mix

Place cream cheese in bowl. Gradually add yogurt. Mix in dressing mix and blend well, using mixer or wire whip. Good as vegetable dip or spread for crackers or bread.

Calories per serving: 37 per 2 tablespoons
Calcium per serving: 40 mg per 2 tablespoons

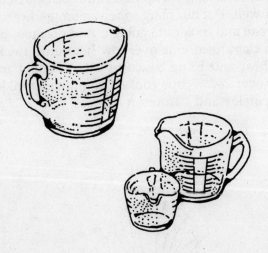

SPICY YOGURT DRESSING

Not for the faint of palate.

Number of servings: Makes about 1¼ cups

> **1 cup plain yogurt**
> **2 tablespoons lemon juice**
> **1 tablespoon sugar**
> **½ cup nonfat dry milk**
> **½ teaspoon salt**
> **⅛–¼ teaspoon ground cumin**
> **⅛ teaspoon black pepper**
> **⅛ teaspoon cayenne pepper**

Put the yogurt in a small mixing bowl. Beat with a fork until smooth and creamy. Stir in the lemon juice, sugar and dry milk until smooth. Blend in the salt, cumin, black pepper and cayenne pepper. Refrigerate in a covered container.

Calories per serving: 32 per 2 tablespoons
Calcium per serving: 84 mg per 2 tablespoons

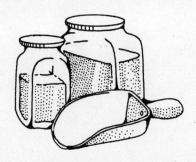

SPINACH SPREAD

A favorite in the Fredal household.

Number of servings: Makes 3 cups

> 2 10-ounce packages frozen chopped spinach,
> thawed and squeezed dry
> ½ cup diet mayonnaise
> 1½ cups plain yogurt
> 1 package Knorr vegetable soup mix
> 2 green onions, finely chopped

Mix all ingredients thoroughly by hand, or use food processor with on/off method. Refrigerate overnight before serving, to blend flavors.

Calories per serving: 25 per 2 tablespoons
Calcium per serving: 49 mg per 2 tablespoons

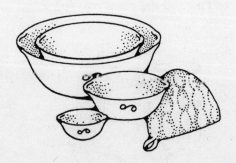

TAHINI DIPPING SAUCE

Sesame-seed paste can be purchased in Middle Eastern or health-food stores.

Number of servings: Makes about 1½ cups

> **5 cloves garlic, finely minced**
> **1 teaspoon salt**
> **½ cup sesame seed paste**
> **½ cup lemon juice**
> **¼ cup cold water**

Crush garlic and salt into a paste. Beat this paste and sesame seed paste in a small bowl with a fork. Add lemon juice and water, one at a time, beating continuously until blended.

Calories per serving: 62 per 2 tablespoons
Calcium per serving: 27 mg per 2 tablespoons

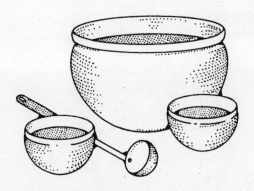

TANGY CHEESE SAUCE

Number of servings: Makes about 2 cups

> **1 tablespoon margarine**
> **1 tablespoon cornstarch**
> **1 teaspoon prepared mustard**
> **¼ teaspoon salt**
> **dash pepper**
> **1¼ cups nonfat milk**
> **4 ounces low-calorie processed cheddar cheese, diced**
> **5 drops red pepper sauce**

Heat margarine over low heat until melted. Blend in cornstarch, mustard, salt and pepper. Cook, stirring constantly, until mixture is smooth; remove from heat. Stir in milk. Heat over low flame until thickened, stirring constantly. Stir in cheese and red pepper sauce. Cook and stir until cheese is melted. Serve over steamed broccoli or cauliflower, or over warm cornbread.

Calories per serving: 29 per 2 tablespoons
Calcium per serving: 78 mg per 2 tablespoons

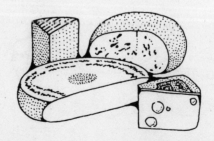

YOGURT CHEESE

A great low-calorie substitute for cream cheese! Plain or sweetened, yogurt cheese goes well with fresh fruit or as a spread for bagels or muffins. Savory variety goes well with bread or crackers.

Number of servings: Makes ½ cup

1 cup plain lowfat yogurt

Flavorings (optional)
Savory:
    ½ tablespoon finely minced parsley
    ⅛ teaspoon salt
    ½ tablespoon finely sliced chives
Sweet:
    **1 tablespoon apple butter or orange marma-
      lade**

Place yogurt in the middle of a triple-thickness square of cheesecloth, large enough to be hung. Bring the four corners of the cheesecloth together and tie. Suspend the bundle where it can drip. (It can be tied to the faucet of the kitchen sink.) Let it drip for 8 hours. Remove resulting cheese into a closed plastic container and refrigerate until eaten. If flavorings are added, mix them into yogurt cheese before refrigeration.

Calories per serving: Savory—18 per tablespoon
                            Sweet—22 per tablespoon
Calcium per serving: 52 mg per tablespoon

WHITE WINE SAUCE

Excellent for poached fish.

Number of servings: Makes 1 cup

> 1 tablespoon margarine
> 2 small shallots, minced
> 1 tablespoon cornstarch
> ⅓ cup dry white wine
> ⅔ cup nonfat evaporated milk
> ¼ teaspoon salt
> ⅛ teaspoon white pepper

Melt margarine in a small saucepan. Add shallots and cook until lightly browned. Stir in cornstarch. Add wine, milk, salt and pepper. Cook over low heat until thickened, stirring constantly. Do not boil. When the sauce is of desired consistency, turn up heat and bring to a light boil; then remove from heat.

Calories per serving: 42 per 2 tablespoons
Calcium per serving: 67 mg per 2 tablespoons

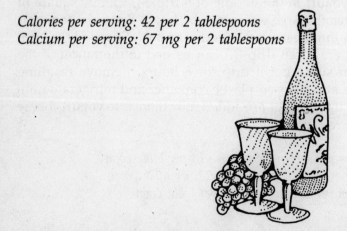

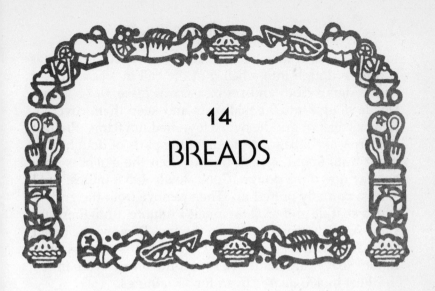

14
BREADS

HEARTY FLAT BREAD

One version of an Indian staple, this bread will complement a thick soup or chowder.

Number of servings: 9 small loaves

> 1⅔ cups whole-wheat flour
> 1⅔ cups all-purpose flour
> 1½ teaspoons double-acting baking powder
> ½ teaspoon salt
> ½ cup nonfat dry milk
> 1¾ cups plain yogurt

Sift the flours, baking powder, salt and dry milk into a bowl. With hands slowly mix in as much yogurt as needed to make a soft, resilient dough. Knead about 10–15 minutes and form dough into a ball. Put the ball in a bowl, cover with a damp cloth and set in a warm place 1½–2 hours. Divide dough into 9 equal parts and keep them covered. Heat a skillet or griddle over a low-medium flame. Preheat broiler. Make a ball out of one of the parts of dough. Roll it out until about ⅛ inch thick. When the skillet is very hot, lay down the dough. Cook slowly 4–5 minutes, until at least partially puffed up. Then remove from the griddle with a spatula and broil for about 1 minute, until there are a few reddish-brown spots on the top. Remove the bread and cover with a clean cloth. Continue this process until all nine loaves are made. To reheat the bread, wrap in foil and heat in 400-degree oven for 15 minutes.

Calories per serving: 201 per loaf
Calcium per serving: 175 mg per bread

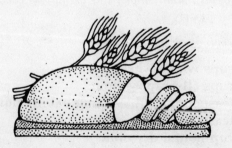

ALMOND-FRUIT BREAD

Number of servings: 16 slices

¼ cup margarine, softened
½ cup sugar
2 teaspoons grated lemon peel
½ teaspoon cinnamon
2 eggs
3 tablespoons nonfat milk
1 teaspoon lemon juice
1⅔ cups flour
½ cup nonfat dry milk
1½ teaspoons baking powder
1 teaspoon salt
¼ teaspoon baking soda
1½ cups peeled shredded apple
1 cup chopped dried figs
½ cup chopped almonds

Cream margarine, sugar, lemon peel and cinnamon. Add eggs and beat until light and fluffy. Beat in milk and lemon juice. Stir remaining dry ingredients together thoroughly and add to creamed mixture until moistened. Fold in apples, figs and almonds. Pour into greased 9×5×3-inch pan and bake at 350 degrees for 1 hour or until toothpick inserted in center comes out clean.

Calories per serving: 171 per 1 slice
Calcium per serving: 61 mg per 1 slice

APPLE-OAT BRAN MUFFINS

Oat bran, a soluble fiber, helps to lower blood-sugar and cholesterol levels.

Number of servings: 12 muffins

> 1 cup whole-wheat flour
> 1½ cups oat bran
> 2½ teaspoons baking powder
> 1 teaspoon salt
> ¼ teaspoon baking soda
> ¼ cup brown sugar, packed
> ½ cup nonfat dry milk
> 1 teaspoon cinnamon
> ½ teaspoon nutmeg
> 3 tablespoons vegetable oil
> 1 cup plain yogurt
> 1 egg
> ¾ cup unsweetened applesauce

In a large bowl, mix flour, oat bran, baking powder, salt, baking soda, sugar, dry milk, cinnamon and nutmeg together thoroughly. In a separate bowl beat oil, yogurt and egg together. Blend in applesauce. Add wet ingredients to dry and blend just until moistened; do not overmix. Grease bottom of muffin pan; pour batter into pan. Bake at 400 degrees for 20 minutes.

Calories per serving: 158
Calcium per serving: 141 mg

CORNBREAD

Number of servings: 16 2¼-inch squares

> **2 cups corn meal**
> ½ **cup whole-wheat flour**
> ½ **cup all-purpose flour**
> ½ **cup nonfat dry milk**
> **4 teaspoons baking powder**
> ¼ **teaspoon baking soda**
> ½ **teaspoon salt**
> **1 egg**
> 1¼ **cups nonfat milk**
> ¼ **cup oil**
> ½ **cup honey**
> **1 teaspoon vanilla**

Sift together corn meal, flours, dry milk, baking powder, baking soda and salt in a large bowl. Beat egg, milk, oil, honey and vanilla. Add to dry ingredients, stirring just enough to moisten. Do not overbeat. Pour into greased 9-inch-square pan and bake at 375 degrees for 30–35 minutes or until golden.

Calories per serving: 173
Calcium per serving: 112 mg

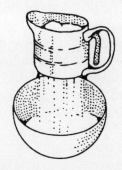

CURRANT SCONES

English cousin to a biscuit, the richer scone dresses up any Sunday brunch.

Number of servings: 12 scones

1⅔ cups all-purpose flour
2 tablespoons sugar
2½ teaspoons baking powder
½ cup nonfat dry milk
½ teaspoon salt
¼ cup margarine
2 eggs, beaten
⅓ cup nonfat evaporated milk
⅓ cup currants

Sift together flour, sugar, baking powder, dry milk and salt. Cut margarine into these ingredients with a pastry blender or two knives until margarine is the size of small peas. Reserve 1 tablespoon of the beaten egg. To the rest, beat in evaporated milk. Make a well in the dry ingredients; pour the liquid and currants into it. Combine the ingredients in swift strokes with a fork until dough is fairly free from the sides of the bowl.

Turn dough onto a lightly floured board and roll it with a lightly floured rolling pin until it is ¾ inch thick. With a floured knife cut dough into diamond shapes. Place them on an ungreased cookie sheet. Brush with the reserved egg and bake in a preheated oven at 425 degrees until golden, about 12–15 minutes.

Calories per serving: 146
Calcium per serving: 120 mg

IRISH SODA LOAF

This quick and easy bread not only is delicious, but brings an old-fashioned aroma to today's busy kitchen.

Number of servings: 16 slices

> **3 tablespoons margarine, softened**
> **2 cups all-purpose flour**
> **²/₃ cup nonfat dry milk**
> **1 teaspoon baking soda**
> **1 teaspoon baking powder**
> **¹/₂ teaspoon salt**
> **2 tablespoons sugar**
> **¹/₃ cup raisins**
> **1 cup plain yogurt**

Cut margarine into flour, dry milk, baking soda, baking powder, salt and sugar until mixture resembles fine crumbs. Stir in raisins and enough yogurt to make a soft dough. Turn onto lightly floured surface; knead until smooth, 1–2 minutes. Shape into round loaf, about 6½ inches in diameter. Place on greased cookie sheet. Cut an X about one-fourth deep in the loaf with floured knife. Bake at 375 degrees until golden brown, about 35 minutes.

Calories per serving: 110
Calcium per serving: 70 mg

PANCAKES À L'ORANGE

Number of servings: 4 pancakes

> **5 tablespoons whole-wheat flour**
> **3 tablespoons nonfat dry milk**
> **1 teaspoon baking powder**
> **dash salt**
> **½ orange, sectioned and finely cut (include juice)**
> **6 tablespoons orange juice**

Sift first four ingredients into mixing bowl. Stir in orange sections and orange juice until dry ingredients are moistened. Spoon batter for four pancakes onto preheated nonstick griddle or pan. Cook over medium heat until golden; flip and brown the other side.

Calories per serving: 62 per pancake
Calcium per serving: 104 mg per pancake

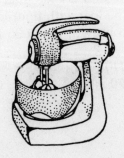

PUMPKIN BREAD

Number of servings: 32 slices

⅓ cup oil
2 cups brown sugar
1 teaspoon vanilla
4 eggs
1 1-pound can pumpkin
1 cup nonfat milk
3⅓ cups flour
1 cup nonfat dry milk
2 teaspoons baking soda
1½ teaspoons salt
½ teaspoon baking powder
1 teaspoon cinnamon
1 teaspoon pumpkin pie spice
1 teaspoon cloves
½ cup raisins

Combine oil and brown sugar in a large bowl. Add vanilla, eggs, pumpkin and milk. Blend in flour, dry milk, baking soda, salt, baking powder, cinnamon, pumpkin pie spice and cloves. Stir in raisins. Pour into two greased 9 × 5 × 3-inch pans. Bake at 350 degrees for about 70 minutes, until toothpick inserted in center comes out clean. Cool slightly before removing from pans.

Calories per serving: 151
Calcium per serving: 59 mg

STRAWBERRY-CHEESE CRÊPES

Sunday morning at Judy's house often meant Dad's delicious crêpes. This version is filled with cottage cheese for extra calcium and protein.

Number of servings: 8 9-inch crêpes

1½ cups low-fat milk
1 tablespoon margarine
3 eggs, beaten
1 cup flour
½ teaspoon salt
vegetable oil spray
2 cups crushed strawberries, fresh or frozen, thawed
1 teaspoon sugar
1 cup low-fat cottage cheese

Heat milk and margarine in a saucepan until margarine melts. When cooled, transfer mixture to a mixing bowl and add eggs, flour and salt, and beat with a hand mixer until smooth. Spray a nonstick skillet with vegetable oil spray and heat. Pour in enough batter to coat the skillet. (Tilt skillet to get the batter coated evenly around the sides.) Cook until browned, about 1 minute. Turn and brown the other side. Remove crêpe from skillet, place on a hot platter and pour more batter into the skillet. Prepare all of the crêpes this way. Sprinkle strawberries with sugar. Spread 1½–2 tablespoons cottage cheese over each crêpe, and roll. Top with 2–3 tablespoons strawberries.

Calories per serving: 213 for 1 crêpe
Calcium per serving: 106 mg for 1 crêpe

WHOLE-GRAIN MUFFINS

High in fiber and complex carbohydrate, one of these muffins and a frothy breakfast shake will start your day out right.

Number of servings: 12 muffins

>   2½ cups whole-wheat flake cereal
>   1½ cups nonfat milk
>   1 egg
>   ⅓ cup vegetable oil
>   1½ cups sifted whole-wheat flour
>   ½ cup sugar
>   ½ cup nonfat dry milk
>   4½ teaspoons baking powder
>   1 teaspoon salt

Combine cereal and milk in mixing bowl. Let stand about 5 minutes, or until cereal is softened. Add egg and oil and beat well. Sift together remaining ingredients. Add to cereal mixture and stir only until moistened. (It will be lumpy.) Fill greased muffin pan. Bake at 375 degrees for 30 minutes or until muffins are lightly browned. Remove immediately.

Calories per serving: 187
Calcium per serving: 123 mg

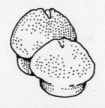

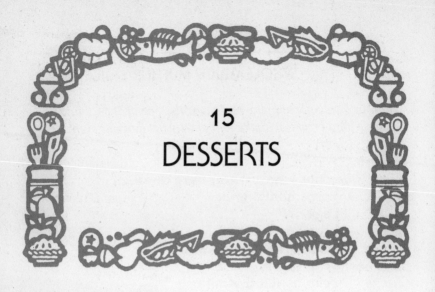

15
DESSERTS

ALMOND COFFEE CAKE

Number of servings: 16

> 1 cup sugar
> ⅓ cup margarine, softened
> 3 eggs
> 1½ teaspoons vanilla
> 1 12-ounce can almond filling
> 3 cups whole-wheat flour
> 2 teaspoons baking powder
> ½ cup nonfat dry milk
> 1½ teaspoons baking soda
> ½ teaspoon salt
> 1½ cups plain yogurt
> 7 tablespoons powdered sugar
> 2 teaspoons warm milk

Grease tube or Bundt cake pan. Beat sugar, margarine, eggs and vanilla in large mixing bowl on medium speed for about 2 minutes, scraping bowl occasionally. Blend in almond filling. Combine flour, baking powder, dry milk, baking soda and salt; blend into egg mixture alternately with yogurt. Pour batter into pan and bake in preheated oven at 350 degrees about 1 hour, until toothpick inserted near center comes out clean. Cool in pan about 15 minutes, then remove from pan. Combine powdered sugar and warm milk until smooth. Drizzle over cake.

Calories per serving: 315
Calcium per serving: 141 mg

COTTAGE CHEESECAKE

Serve with fresh strawberries or other fruit topping.

Number of servings: 12

Crust:
20 graham cracker squares
4 tablespoons margarine, softened
2 tablespoons sugar

Filling:
2 pounds low-fat cottage cheese, drained
3/4 cup sugar
3 eggs, lightly beaten
1 teaspoon vanilla

Topping:
   1 cup plain yogurt, drained of excess liquid (if
      firm topping is desired, hang yogurt in tri-
      ple-layered cheesecloth for 1–2 hours to re-
      move excess liquid)
   2½ tablespoons sugar
   1½ teaspoons vanilla

To make pie crust, crush graham crackers with rolling pin, or in blender or food processor. Mix in margarine and sugar until fine crumbs are made. Press mixture into the bottom of a 9-inch springform pan. Bake at 350 degrees for 10 minutes.

To make the filling, blend cottage cheese, sugar, eggs and vanilla in blender or food processor until smooth. Pour into pie crust and bake at 350 degrees until firm, about 40 minutes.

To make the topping, blend yogurt, sugar and vanilla. Spread over baked cheesecake and let cool. Refrigerate before serving.

Calories per serving: 245
Calcium per serving: 100 mg

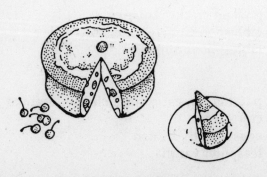

EASY YOGURT PIE

Number of servings: 6

> 2 cups (2 cartons) low-fat fruit yogurt (straw-
> berry, blueberry, etc.)
> ½ cup crushed fruit (same kind as the yogurt),
> fresh or frozen (unsweetened) and thawed
> 6 ounces evaporated whole milk, chilled
> 1 teaspoon lemon juice
> 2 tablespoons sugar
> 1 teaspoon vanilla
> 1 graham cracker pie crust
>
> *Also needed:*
> chilled metal bowl
> chilled beaters

In a bowl, blend yogurt and fruit well. Pour milk into
chilled bowl and beat with chilled beaters until foamy. Add
lemon juice and beat until firm; add sugar and vanilla and
beat until stiff. Fold whipped milk thoroughly into yogurt
mixture. Spoon into crust and freeze about 4 hours. Remove from freezer and place in refrigerator for 30 minutes
before serving (or longer for softer texture). Store in freezer.

Calories per serving: 316
Calcium per serving: 211 mg

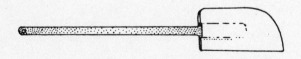

FROZEN ORANGE YOGURT

This is as good as the soft-serve kind, and easy to make at home.

Number of servings: 9 1-cup servings

> **1 3-ounce package orange-flavored gelatin**
> **¾ cup sugar**
> **1 cup water**
> **1 cup orange juice**
> **2 cups plain yogurt**
> **1 cup evaporated whole milk, chilled**
> *Also needed:*
> **2 chilled metal bowls (2 sizes)**
> **chilled beaters**

Combine gelatin, sugar and water in saucepan. Boil, stirring constantly, until sugar and gelatin are dissolved. Remove from heat and cool to room temperature (about 30 minutes). Stir in orange juice and yogurt. Pour into 9 × 13-inch pan. Freeze, stirring occasionally, until partially frozen, 2–3 hours. Spoon into chilled large bowl. Beat with chilled beaters until very smooth. In a smaller chilled bowl, whip milk until stiff. Fold whipped milk into yogurt mixture. Spoon into bowl or freezer container; cover and freeze until firm, 3–4 hours.

Calories per serving: 181
Calcium per serving: 168 mg

PEACH POPSICLES

A light, summery treat . . . good anytime of the year!

Number of servings: 12 popsicles

> **20 ounces frozen sweetened peaches (if unsweet-
> ened peaches are used, add 4 tablespoons
> sugar to juice)
> reserved peach juice from frozen peaches
> 1 envelope unflavored gelatin
> 2 cups plain yogurt**
> *Also needed:*
> **12 3-ounce paper cups
> 12 wooden popsicle sticks**

Thaw peaches completely. Press thoroughly to remove all juice. Place drained juice (and sugar, if used) in a saucepan and sprinkle with gelatin. Cook over low heat, stirring until gelatin dissolves. Blend peaches, yogurt and juice with gelatin in a blender until smooth. Place cups in a baking pan and fill with fruit mixture. Cover each cup with waxed paper; make a slit in the paper over the center of each cup and insert a stick for each popsicle. Freeze until firm. Run warm water on outside of cup to loosen it from popsicle before serving.

Calories per serving: 73
Calcium per serving: 70 mg

FRUIT-'N'-SPICE RICE PUDDING

Not too sweet, this pudding makes a nice afternoon or evening snack.

Number of servings: 16 ½-cup servings

- ⅔ cup nonfat dry milk
- 3⅓ cups nonfat milk
- 2 cups uncooked white rice
- pinch salt
- ⅔ cup honey
- 2 eggs, beaten
- 1 teaspoon cinnamon
- ½ teaspoon powdered ginger
- 2 cups coarsely chopped oranges
- 1 cup orange- or vanilla-flavored yogurt

Blend dry milk with liquid milk until smooth. Heat milk, rice and salt to near boiling, stirring once or twice; reduce heat. Cover and simmer for 14 minutes; do not stir. When cooked the rice should be tender but will be wet. Remove from heat. Stir in honey, eggs, cinnamon and ginger. Spread a third of rice mixture over bottom of greased 1½-quart casserole. Carefully spread 1 cup orange chunks over rice. Repeat the two layers and top with the last third of rice. Bake in preheated oven at 350 degrees for 25 minutes. Remove from oven; cool slightly. Chill several hours before serving. Top each serving with yogurt.

Calories per serving: 193
Calcium per serving: 150 mg

PRUNE WHIP

Number of servings: 8 ½ cup servings

> 1 cup cut-up cooked prunes (remove pits)
> 3 egg whites
> ⅓ cup sugar
> ½ teaspoon cinnamon
> ¼ teaspoon salt
> 1 tablespoon lemon juice
> ¼ cup chopped hazelnuts

Whipped Topping:
> 1 cup evaporated nonfat milk, chilled
> 1 tablespoon lemon juice
> 3 tablespoons sugar
> 1 teaspoon vanilla

Also needed:
> chilled metal bowl
> chilled beaters

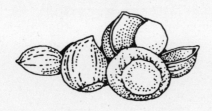

Blend prunes in food processor or blender until smooth. In a mixing bowl beat prunes, egg whites, sugar, cinnamon and salt until stiff. Fold in lemon juice and hazelnuts. Pour into ungreased 1½-quart casserole. Place casserole in pan on oven rack. Pour very hot water, 1 inch deep, into pan. Bake uncovered in 350-degree oven until puffed and thin film has formed on top, 30 to 35 minutes. Serve warm with whipped topping.

Whipped topping: Pour milk into chilled bowl and beat with chilled beaters until foamy. Add lemon juice and beat until firm. Add sugar and vanilla and beat until stiff. Whipped milk will hold its shape for up to 1 hour, if re-frigerated.

Calories per serving: 131
Calcium per serving: 108 mg

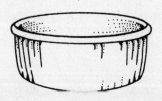

PUMPKIN CUSTARD

Number of servings: 6

> ½ **cup nonfat dry milk**
> 1 **12-ounce can nonfat evaporated milk**
> 3 **eggs, slightly beaten**
> ½ **cup brown sugar**
> 1 **1-pound can pumpkin**
> 1 **teaspoon salt**
> 1 **teaspoon cinnamon**
> ½ **teaspoon ginger**
> ½ **teaspoon cloves**
>   **nutmeg**

Heat oven to 350 degrees. Blend dry milk into evaporated milk. Mix together eggs, sugar, pumpkin, salt, cinnamon, ginger and cloves. Stir in milk gradually. Pour into six 6-ounce custard cups; sprinkle with nutmeg. Place cups in 9 × 13-inch pan on oven rack. Pour very hot water into pan to within ½ inch of top of cups. Bake until knife inserted halfway between center and edge comes out clean, about 45 minutes. Remove cups from water. Serve warm or chilled.

Calories per serving: 205
Calcium per serving: 304 mg

SPECIAL BAKED APPLE

Number of servings: 2

> **1 large apple**
> **¼ teaspoon cinnamon**
> **1 tablespoon packed brown sugar**
> **1 cup plain yogurt**

Core and slice apple; arrange in small casserole. Top with cinnamon and brown sugar. Bake uncovered at 375 degrees until tender, about 40 minutes. After 20 minutes, stir slices. Transfer slices to serving dishes and top each with ½ cup plain yogurt.

Calories per serving: 164
Calcium per serving: 222 mg

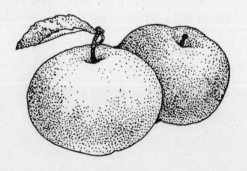

YOGURT FRUIT PUDDING

Number of servings: 4 1-cup servings

> **2 cups strawberries, fresh or frozen (unsweetened)**
> **1 cup cold nonfat milk**
> **1 cup strawberry yogurt**
> **1 3½-ounce package instant vanilla pudding mix**

Slice strawberries, saving four. If frozen strawberries are used, thaw and drain before slicing. Line bottom of four dessert cups with strawberry slices. Combine milk and yogurt in mixing bowl. Add vanilla pudding mix and beat slowly until blended, about 2 minutes. Let stand until set, about 5 minutes. Dish pudding into dessert cups and top with whole strawberries.

Calories per serving: 220
Calcium per serving: 263 mg

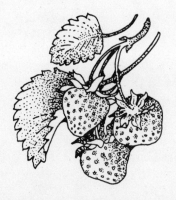

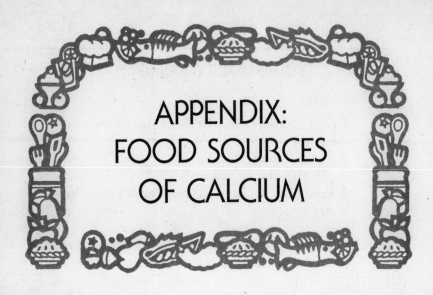

APPENDIX: FOOD SOURCES OF CALCIUM

SOURCE	CALCIUM (mg)	CALORIES
Dairy		
Buttermilk, 1 cup	285	99
Cheese, 1 oz.		
American	174	106
Blue	150	100
Brick	191	105
Cheddar	204	114
Colby	194	112
Edam	207	101
Feta	140	75
Gouda	198	101
Gruyère	287	117
Monterey Jack	212	106
Mozzarella, part-skim	183	72
Muenster	203	104
Parmesan	336	111

SOURCE	CALCIUM (mg)	CALORIES
Provolone	214	100
Romano	302	110
Swiss	272	107
Cheese, low-fat, American, 1 slice (²/₃ oz.)	134	34
Cheese food, American, 1 oz.	163	93
Cheese food, Swiss, 1 oz.	205	92
Cheese, ricotta, ½ cup	257	216
Cheese, ricotta, part-skim, ½ cup	337	171
Cheese spread, American, 1 oz.	159	82
Cocoa, from mix, 1 cup	107	110
Cottage cheese, creamed, ½ cup	63	117
Cottage cheese, 2% low-fat, ½ cup	77	101
Ice cream, vanilla, 10% fat, 1 cup	176	269
Ice cream, vanilla, soft-serve, 1 cup	236	377
Ice milk, vanilla, 1 cup	176	184
Milk		
evaporated, nonfat, ½ cup	368	100
evaporated, whole, ½ cup	328	168
low-fat (1%), 1 cup	300	102
low-fat (2%), 1 cup	297	121
nonfat, 1 cup	302	86
nonfat, dry, instant, ⅓ cup	280	82

SOURCE	CALCIUM (mg)	CALORIES
whole, 1 cup	291	150
whole, chocolate, 1 cup	284	208
Milk shake, vanilla, 10 oz.	329	352
Pudding, chocolate, from instant, ½ cup	150	179
Pudding, sugar-free, from instant, ½ cup	161	65
Whipped evaporated milk, whole, 2 tbsp.	27	14
Yogurt, low-fat, vanilla, 1 cup	389	194
Yogurt, low-fat, fruited, 1 cup	345	231
Yogurt, plain, lowfat, 1 cup	415	144

Proteins

Almonds, ¼ cup	83	221
Anchovies, canned, 8 fillets	47	49
Beans, dried, cooked, ½ cup		
Chickpeas (garbanzo beans)	40	134
Great northern beans	60	104
Navy (pea) beans	64	129
Pinto beans	41	117
Soybeans	88	149
Brazil nuts, ¼ cup	65	226
Clams, 3½ oz., 5 large	69	80
Clams, canned, ½ cup	55	52
Egg, scrambled with milk, 1 large	47	85
Filberts (hazelnuts), ¼ cup	71	181

SOURCE	CALCIUM (mg)	CALORIES
Herring, canned, 3½ oz.	147	208
Lobster, northern, canned, ½ cup	55	75
Mackerel, Pacific, canned, 3½ oz.	260	180
Mussels, 3½ oz.	88	95
Oysters, eastern, raw, 5–8 medium	94	66
Salmon, canned with bones, 3½ oz.	154	210
Sardines, canned in oil, 3½ oz., 8 medium	354	311
Sardines, canned in tomato sauce, 3½ oz.	449	230
Scallops, 3½ oz.	115	112
Sesame seeds, decorticated, 1 oz.	35	167
Shrimp, canned, 3½ oz.	115	116
Smelt, canned, 3½ oz., 4–5 medium	358	200
Sole, raw, 3½ oz.	61	68
Sunflower seed kernels, ¼ cup	44	203
Tofu, firm, processed with calcium sulfate, ½ cup	861	183
Tofu, regular, ½ cup, processed		
with added calcium	434	94
without added calcium	130	94

Vegetables

Artichoke, 1 large	51	44

SOURCE	CALCIUM (mg)	CALORIES
Bok choy (white mustard cabbage), cooked, ½ cup	126	12
Broccoli, fresh, cooked, ⅔ cup or 1 large stalk	88	26
Broccoli, frozen, cooked, ⅔ cup	37	27
Broccoli, raw, 1 stalk	103	32
Cabbage, cooked, ½ cup	37	17
Endive, raw, 10 long leaves	41	10
Fennel, raw, 1 cup	67	19
Greens, cooked, ½ cup		
Beet greens	99	18
Collard greens	152	29
Dandelion	140	33
Kale	89	19
Mustard greens	138	23
Spinach	83	21
Swiss chard	61	15
Turnip greens	137	15
Lettuce, romaine, 1 cup	51	14
Okra, frozen, cooked, ½ cup	72	26
Parsley, chopped, 2 tbsp.	40	8
Rhubarb, frozen, raw, 1 cup	266	29
Rutabaga, diced, cooked, ½ cup	59	35
Squash		
acorn, baked, ½ medium	61	86
butternut, baked, 1 cup	82	139

SOURCE	CALCIUM (mg)	CALORIES
hubbard, baked, 1 cup	49	103
Sweet potato, baked,		
1 large	72	254
Watercress, raw, chopped,		
1 cup	151	19
Wax beans, ½ cup	50	22

Fruits

Blackberries, 1 cup	46	74
Boysenberries, 1 cup	46	88
Currants, Zante, dried,		
½ cup	62	204
Elderberries, 1 cup	55	105
Fig, dried, 5	135	239
Indian fig, 3½ oz.	57	67
Mulberries, 1 cup	55	61
Orange, navel, 1 medium	56	65
Papaya, 1 medium	72	117
Prunes, dried, 10	43	201

Grains

Biscuit, 1 small (about 1 oz.		
or 2 inches wide),		
from mix	58	93
Bran muffin, 1 small (1½		
oz.)	54	112
Cornbread, 1 3-oz. piece	90	198
English muffin, 1	92	135
Pancake, 1 large, from mix	96	159
Tortilla, corn, 6-inch		
diameter	60	67
Waffle, 1 frozen	85	86

SOURCE	CALCIUM (mg)	CALORIES
Miscellaneous		
Beans, baked in tomato sauce, canned, ½ cup	82	116
Custard, baked, ½ cup	148	153
Molasses, blackstrap, 1 tbsp.	116	43
Pizza, cheese, ¼ of 12-inch pie	291	326
Soup, cream of chicken, canned, made with milk, 1 cup	180	191
Soup, cream of mushroom, canned, made with milk, 1 cup	178	203

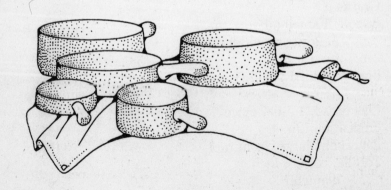

REFERENCES

Allen, L. H. Calcium bioavailability and absorption: A review. *American Journal of Clinical Nutrition* 35(4): 783, 1982.

Calcium supplements—some clinical guidelines. *Nutrition and the M.D.* 12(3):5, 1986.

Fanelli, M. T. Promoting women's health. *Dietetic Currents* 12(4): 19, 1985.

Gordan, G. S., and Vaughan, C. Calcium and osteoporosis. *Journal of Nutrition* 116(2): 319, 1986.

National Dairy Council. *Calcium: A Summary of Current Research for the Health Professional*. Rosemont, Illinois: 1984.

Nilas, J., Christiansen, C., and Rodbro, P. Calcium supplementation and postmenopausal bone loss. *British Medical Journal* 289:1103, 1984.

Pennington, J. A. T., and Church, H. N. *Food Values of Portions Commonly Used* (14th ed.). Philadelphia: Lippincott, 1985.

Quint, L., and Liebman, B. Putting calcium into perspective. *Nutrition Action Healthletter* 14(6):8, 1987.

Riis, B., Thomsen, K., and Christiansen, C. Does calcium supplementation prevent postmenopausal bone loss? A double-blind, controlled clinical study. *New England Journal of Medicine* 316(4): 173, 1987.

Spencer, H. Minerals and mineral interactions in human beings. *Journal of the American Dietetic Association* 86(7): 864, 1986.

Spencer, H., and Kramer, L. Factors contributing to osteoporosis. *Journal of Nutrition* 116(2): 316, 1986.

Tremaine, W. J., et al. Calcium absorption from milk in lactase-deficient and lactase-sufficient adults. *Digest Dis Science* 31(4): 376, 1986.

U.S. Department of Agriculture, Agricultural Research Service. *Composition of Foods, Dairy and Egg Products: Raw, Processed, Prepared.* Washington, D.C.: Superintendent of Documents, U.S. Government Printing Office, Agriculture Handbook No. 8-1, 1976.

U.S. Department of Agriculture, Agricultural Research Service. *Composition of Foods, Legumes and Legume Products: Raw, Processed, Prepared.* Washington, D.C.: Superintendent of Documents, U.S. Government Printing Office, Agriculture Handbook No. 8-16, 1986.

U.S. Department of Agriculture, Agricultural Research Service. *Composition of Foods, Soups, Sauces, and Gravies: Raw, Processed, Prepared.* Washington, D.C.: Superintendent of Documents, U.S. Government Printing Office, Agriculture Handbook No. 8-6, 1980.

U.S. Department of Agriculture, Agricultural Research Service. *Nutritive Value of American Foods in Common Units.* Washington, D.C.: Superintendent of Documents, U.S. Government Printing Office, Agriculture Handbook No. 456, 1975.

INDEX

INDEX

INDEX

INDEX

INDEX

INDEX

INDEX